Lenore Manderson, PhD, FASSA
Editor

Teaching Gender, Teaching Women's Health: Case Studies in Medical and Health Science Education

Teaching Gender, Teaching Women's Health: Case Studies in Medical and Health Science Education has been co-published simultaneously as *Women & Health*, Volume 37, Number 4 2003.

Pre-publication
REVIEWS,
COMMENTARIES,
EVALUATIONS . . .

"WILL BENEFIT ALL MEDICAL AND HEALTH SCIENCE EDUCATORS. . . . Contributes valuable perspectives on many of the challenges that remain in achieving the goal of equity."

Janet Bickel, MA
President
Janet Bickel & Associates

More pre-publication
REVIEWS, COMMENTARIES, EVALUATIONS . . .

"This book is an antidote to the obstacles encountered when a social construct, such as gender, is championed in the biological world of medicine. Whether it is challenging gender norms and stereotypes, promoting patient autonomy, questioning why an individual is afflicted by a particular illness, or learning shy a focus on women's health, rather than gender, makes men the norm and marginalizes women as 'other,' this book is FULL OF THOUGHT-PROVOKING EXAMPLES OF THE WHYS AND HOWS OF GENDER MAINSTREAMING."

Susan P. Phillips, MD, CCFP, MSc
Associate Professor and Coordinator
Women's Health Program
Queen's University School of Medicine
Kingston, Ontario

"VALUABLE to anyone involved in medical and health science education. . . . Provides much-needed insight. . . . One comes away not only with ideas about how to improve teaching a gender perspective but also a sense of what one can expect to confront in attempting to integrate gender issues into medical curricula. The authors are pioneers in the integration of a gender perspective in medicine and they describe their experiences in quite different settings with a tone that is direct and conversational, which makes this collection TRULY ENJOYABLE TO READ."

Ursula K. Snyder, PhD
Editor/Program Director
Medscape Ob/Gyn & Women's Health
New York City

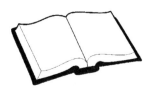

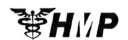

The Haworth Medical Press
An Imprint of The Haworth Press, Inc.

Teaching Gender, Teaching Women's Health: Case Studies in Medical and Health Science Education

Teaching Gender, Teaching Women's Health: Case Studies in Medical and Health Science Education has been co-published simultaneously as *Women & Health*, Volume 37, Number 4 2003.

The *Women & Health* Monographic "Separates"

Below is a list of "separates," which in serials librarianship means a special issue simultaneously published as a special journal issue or double-issue *and* as a "separate" hardbound monograph. (This is a format which we also call a "DocuSerial.")

"Separates" are published because specialized libraries or professionals may wish to purchase a specific thematic issue by itself in a format which can be separately cataloged and shelved, as opposed to purchasing the journal on an on-going basis. Faculty members may also more easily consider a "separate" for classroom adoption.

"Separates" are carefully classified separately with the major book jobbers so that the journal tie-in can be noted on new book order slips to avoid duplicate purchasing.

You may wish to visit Haworth's website at . . .

http://www.HaworthPress.com

. . . to search our online catalog for complete tables of contents of these separates and related publications.

You may also call 1-800-HAWORTH (outside US/Canada: 607-722-5857), or Fax: 1-800-895-0582 (outside US/Canada: 607-771-0012), or e-mail at:

docdelivery@haworthpress.com

Teaching Gender, Teaching Women's Health: Case Studies in Medical and Health Science Education, edited by Lenore Manderson, PhD, FASSA (Vol. 37, No. 4, 2003). *"VALUABLE to anyone involved in medical and health science education. . . . Provides much-needed insight." (Ursula K. Snyder, PhD, Editor/Program Director, Medscape Ob/Gyn & Women's Health, New York City)*

Environmental, Policy and Cultural Factors Related to Physical Activity in a Diverse Sample of Women: The Women's Cardiovascular Health Network Project, edited by Amy A. Eyler, PhD (Vol. 36, No. 2, 2002). *"INTERESTING AND UNIQUE. . . . A MUST-READ for anyone interested in designing, implementing, and evaluating physical activity interventions for underserved–and typically inactive–women." (Lynda Randsell, PhD, FACSM, Assistant Professor of Exercise & Sport Science, University of Utah-Salt Lake City)*

Women's Health in Mainland Southeast Asia, edited by Andrea Whittaker, PhD (Vol. 35, No. 4, 2002). *Shows how war, military regimes, industrialization, urbanization, and social upheaval have all affected the choices Southeast Asian women make about their health and health care.*

Domestic Violence and Health Care: Policies and Prevention, edited by Carolina Reyes, MD, William J. Rudman, PhD, and Calvin R. Hewitt, MBA (Vol. 35, No. 2/3, 2002). *Examines the role of health care in the struggle to combat domestic violence.*

Women's Work, Health and Quality of Life, edited by Afaf Ibrahim Meleis, PhD, FAAN (Vol. 33, No. 1/2, 2001). *"A FINE COLLECTION. . . . A useful supplement for courses on women and health. It is particularly helpful to have a collection that reports research on women in different countries. . . . Describes role overload, role strain, and stress that occurs when immigrants try to adjust to a new culture." (Eleanor Krassen Covan, PhD, Professor of Sociology, Director of Gerontology, University of North Carolina, Wilmington)*

Welfare, Work and Well-Being, edited by Mary Clare Lennon, PhD, MS (Vol. 32, No. 1/2 & No. 3, 2001). *Examines the relationship between social roles, economic circumstances, material hardship, and child well-being among low-income women.*

Australian Women's Health: Innovations in Social Science and Community Research, edited by Lenore Manderson, PhD (Vol. 28, No. 1, 1998). *Reflects a wider approach to women's health, which moves from maternity and fertility issues to question the impact of gender on all aspects of the disease experience.*

Women, Drug Use and HIV Infection, edited by Sally J. Stevens, PhD, Stephanie Tortu, PhD, and Susan L. Coyle, PhD (Vol. 27, No. 1/2, 1998). *"A much-needed resource of critical information about the largest initiative to date designed to prevent HIV among drug users and their sexual partners." (Robert E. Booth, PhD, Associate Professor of Psychiatry, University of Colorado School of Medicine, Denver)*

Women in the Later Years: Health, Social, and Cultural Perspectives, edited by Lois Grau, PhD, RN, in collaboration with Ida Susser, PhD (Vol. 14, No. 3/4, 1989). *"An excellent overview of the pertinent social, political, and personal issues of this long-ignored group." (News for Women in Psychiatry)*

Government Policy and Women's Health Care: The Swedish Alternative, edited by Gunnela Westlander, PhD, and Jeanne Mager Stellman, PhD (Vol. 13, No. 3/4, 1988). *"An illuminating, comprehensive overview of Swedish women's health and their productive and reproductive roles." (Freda L. Paltiel, Senior Advisor, Status of Women, Health and Welfare Canada, Ottawa, Ontario, Canada)*

Embryos, Ethics, and Women's Rights: Exploring the New Reproductive Technologies, edited by Elaine Hoffman Baruch, Amadeo F. D'Adamo, Jr., and Joni Seager (Vol. 13, No. 1/2, 1988). *"Groundbreaking . . . Reveals the myriad of perspectives from which the new technologies can be regarded. Particularly thought-provoking are discussions that link surrogacy to economic and class issues." (Publishers Weekly)*

Women, Health, and Poverty (also published as Dealing with the Health Needs of Women in Poverty), edited by Cesar A. Perales and Lauren S. Young, EdD (Vol. 12, No. 3/4, 1988). *"Succeeds in alerting readers to many important issues. . . Should be useful to public policymakers, researchers, and others interested in understanding the health problems of poor women." (Contemporary Psychology)*

Women and Cancer, edited by Steven D. Stellman, PhD (Vol. 11, No. 3/4, 1987). *"The contributors succeed in increasing the reader's awareness of cancer in women and in stimulating thought processes in reference to the need for further research." (Oncology Nursing Forum)*

Health Needs of Women as They Age, edited by Sharon Golub, PhD, and Rita Jackaway Freedman, PhD (Vol. 10, No. 2/3, 1985). *"The contributors distill a great deal of general information on aging into an easily readable and understandable format . . . A useful primer." (The New England Journal of Medicine)*

Health Care of the Female Adolescent, edited by Sharon Golub, PhD (Vol. 9, No. 2/3, 1985). *"An excellent collection of well-written and carefully selected articles designed to provide up-to-date information about the health problems of adolescent girls." (Journal of the American Medical Women's Association)*

Lifting the Curse of Menstruation: A Feminist Appraisal of the Influence of Menstruation on Women's Lives, edited by Sharon Golub, PhD (Vol. 8, No. 2/3, 1983). *"Crammed with information and well-documented. Written in a professional style, each chapter is followed by extensive lists of notes and references." (Journal of Sex Education and Therapy)*

Obstetrical Intervention and Technology in the 1980s, edited by Diony Young, BA (Vol. 7, No. 3/4, 1983). *"Every family physician and obstetrician in North America should read this book." (Canadian Family Physician)*

Teaching Gender, Teaching Women's Health: Case Studies in Medical and Health Science Education

Lenore Manderson, PhD, FASSA
Editor

Teaching Gender, Teaching Women's Health: Case Studies in Medical and Health Science Education has been co-published simultaneously as *Women & Health*, Volume 37, Number 4 2003.

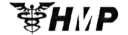

The Haworth Medical Press®
An Imprint of The Haworth Press, Inc.

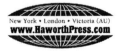

New York • London • Victoria (AU)
www.HaworthPress.com

Published by

The Haworth Medical Press®, 10 Alice Street, Binghamton, NY 13904-1580 USA

The Haworth Medical Press® is an imprint of The Haworth Press, Inc., 10 Alice Street, Binghamton, NY 13904-1580 USA.

Teaching Gender, Teaching Women's Health: Case Studies in Medical and Health Science Education has been co-published simultaneously as *Women & Health*, Volume 37, Number 4 2003.

Cover design by Jennifer M. Gaska

'New York Medical College for Women,' wood engraved print, Frank Leslie's illustrated newspaper, New York, 1870. Courtesy of the National Library of Medicine.

Library of Congress Cataloging-in-Publication Data

Manderson, Lenore.
   Teaching gender, teaching women's health: case studies in medical and health science education / Lenore Manderson.
       p. cm.
   "Teaching and Gender has been co-published simultaneously as Women & Health, Volume 37, Number 4 2003."
   Includes bibliographical references and index.
   ISBN 0-7890-2243-5 (hc : alk. paper)–ISBN 0-7890-2244-3 (alk. paper)
   1. Women physicians–Education. 2. Sex differences in education. 3. Women–Health and hygiene. 4. Women in medicine. 5. Sex discrimination in medical education. 6. Medical education. I. Title.
R692.M325 2003
610'.82–dc21

                                                                                          2003011618

Indexing, Abstracting & Website/Internet Coverage

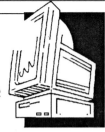

This section provides you with a list of major indexing & abstracting services. That is to say, each service began covering this periodical during the year noted in the right column. Most Websites which are listed below have indicated that they will either post, disseminate, compile, archive, cite or alert their own Website users with research-based content from this work. (This list is as current as the copyright date of this publication.)

Abstracting, Website/Indexing Coverage . . . . Year When Coverage Began

- *Abstracts in Anthropology* **1991**
- *Abstracts in Social Gerontology: Current Literature on Aging* **1991**
- *Academic Abstracts/CD-ROM* **1992**
- *Academic ASAP <www.galegroup.com>* **1988**
- *Academic Search: database of 2,000 selected academic serials, updated monthly: EBSCO Publishing* **1995**
- *Academic Search Elite (EBSCO)* **1993**
- *Academic Search Premier (EBSCO)* **1993**
- *Behavioral Medicine Abstracts* **1996**
- *Biology Digest (in print & online)* **1991**
- *Biosciences Information Service of Biological Abstracts (BIOSIS) a centralized source of life science information <www.biosis.org>* . . . . . ***
- *Cambridge Scientific Abstracts (Health & Safety Science Abstracts/Risk Abstracts) <www.csa.com>* **2001**
- *CINAHL (Cumulative Index to Nursing & Allied Health Literature) <www.cinahl.com>* **1985**
- *CNPIEC Reference Guide: Chinese National Directory of Foreign Periodicals* **1995**
- *Combined Health Information Database (CHID)* **1994**
- *Contemporary Women's Issues* **1998**

(continued)

- *Criminal Justice Abstracts* 1990
- *Current Contents/Social & Behavioral Sciences*
  <www.isinet.com>....................................... 1995
- *Educational Research Abstracts (ERA) (online database)*
  <www.tandf.co.uk>...................................... 2001
- *EMBASE/Excerpta Medica Secondary Publishing Division*
  <URL: http://www.elsevier.nl>............................ 1988
- *Environmental Sciences and Pollution Management (Cambridge*
  Scientific Abstracts Internet Database Service) <www.csa.com> ..... *
- *e-psyche, LLC <www.e-psyche.net>* 2001
- *Expanded Academic ASAP <www.galegroup.com>* 1988
- *Expanded Academic ASAP–International <www.galegroup.com>* ... 1988
- *Family Index Database <www.familyscholar.com>* 2000
- *Family & Society Studies Worldwide <www.nisc.com>*........... 1986
- *Family Violence & Sexual Assault Bulletin*.................... 1999
- *Feminist Periodicals: A Current Listing of Contents* 1982
- *GenderWatch <www.slinfo.com>* 1998
- *General Science Abstracts. Published by The H W Wilson*
  Company <www.hwwilson.com> 1992
- *General Science Index <www.hwwilson.com>*................... 1994
- *General Science Plus Text database, available on ProQuest*
  Information & Learning <www.proquest.com> 1992
- *General Science Source: comprehensive abstracts of nearly*
  200 general science periodicals, updated monthly: EBSCO
  Publishing... 1995
- *Health Management Information Service (HELMIS)*............. 1995
- *Health Reference Center <www.galegroup.com>* 1996
- *Health Reference Center–Academic <www.galegroup.com>* 1996
- *Health Source: Indexing & Abstracting of 160 selected health*
  related journals, updated monthly: EBSCO Publishing.......... 1995
- *Health Source: Nursing/Academic Edition: Indexing &*
  Abstracting of nearly 850 selected nursing and health related
  journals: EBSCO Publishing.............................. 1993
- *Health Source Plus: expanded version of "Health Source":*
  EBSCO Publishing...................................... 1995
- *HealthSTAR*... 1996
- *Higher Education Abstracts, providing the latest in research &*
  theory in more than 140 major topics 1992
- *IBZ International Bibliography of Periodical Literature*
  <www.saur.de>... 1996

(continued)

- *Index Guide to College Journals (core list compiled by integrating 48 indexes frequently used to support undergraduate programs in small to medium sized libraries)* 1999
- *Index Medicus (National Library of Medicine) <www.nlm.nih.gov>* ... 1992
- *Index to Periodical Articles Related to Law* 1990
- *Industrial Hygiene Digest* 1996
- *InfoTrac Custom <www.galegroup.com>*........................ 1996
- *MasterFILE: updated database from EBSCO Publishing* 1995
- *MasterFILE Premier: coverage of more than 1,950 periodicals covering general reference, business, health, education, general science, multi-cultural issues and much more: EBSCO Publishing* 1993
- *MasterFILE Select: coverage of nearly 770 periodicals covering general reference, business, health, education, general science, multi-cultural issues and much more: EBSCO Publishing* 1993
- *MEDLINE (National Library of Medicine) <www.nlm.nih.gov>*..... 1992
- *National Center for Chronic Disease Prevention & Health Promotion (NCCDPHP)*................................... 1998
- *NIAAA Alcohol and Alcohol Problems Science Database (ETOH) <http://etoh.niaaa.nih.gov>*....................... 1995
- *OCLC ArticleFirst <http://www.oclc.org/services/databases/>* .... *
- *OCLC ContentsFirst <http://www.oclc.org/services/databases/>* .... *
- *OCLC Public Affairs Information Service <www.pais.org>* 1988
- *OmniFile Full Text: Mega Edition (only available electronically) <www.hwwilson.com>* 1987
- *ONS Nursing Scan in Oncology–NAACOG's Women's Health Nursing Scan* 1996
- *Papillomavirus Report, Leeds Medical Information* 1997
- *PASCAL, c/o Institute de L'Information Scientifique et Technique <http://www.inist.fr>* 1994
- *Periodical Abstracts, Research I (general & basic reference indexing & abstracting data-base from University Microfilms International) (UMI)*........................... 1992
- *Periodical Abstracts, Research II (broad coverage indexing & abstracting data-base from University Microfilms International) (UMI)* 1992
- *Periodical Abstracts Select (abstracting & indexing service covering most frequently requested journals in general reference, plus journals requested in libraries serving undergraduate programs, available from University Microfilms International) (UMI)*........................... 1994

(continued)

- *Physiotherapy Evidence Database (PEDro)*
  <http://ptwww.cchs.usyd.edu.au/pedro> 1999
- *ProQuest 5000 database, available on ProQuest Information &*
  Learning <www.proquest.com> 1992
- *ProQuest Research Library database, available on ProQuest*
  Information & Learning <www.proquest.com> . . . . *
- *POPLINE* 1992
- *Psychological Abstracts (PsycINFO) <www.apa.org>* 1989
- *PubMed (National Library of Medicine) <www.nlm.nih.gov>* 1992
- *Referativnyi Zhurnal (Abstracts Journal of the All-Russian*
  Institute of Scientific and Technical Information–in Russian) . . . 1990
- *RESEARCH ALERT/ISI Alerting Services <www.isinet.com>* 1995
- *Sage Family Studies Abstracts (SFSA)* 1991
- *Social Science Source: coverage of 400 journals in the*
  social sciences area; updated monthly; EBSCO Publishing 1995
- *Social Sciences Abstracts & Social Sciences Full Text*
  <www.hwwilson.com> 1987
- *Social Sciences Citation Index <www.isinet.com>* 1995
- *Social Sciences Index (from Volume 1 & continuing)*
  <www.hwwilson.com> 1976
- *Social Sciences PlusText database, available on ProQuest*
  Information & Learning <www.proquest.com> 1992
- *Social Scisearch <www.isinet.com>* 1995
- *Social Services Abstracts <www.csa.com>* 1992
- *Social Work Abstracts <www.silverplatter.com/catalog/swab.htm>* . . . 1982
- *SocioAbs <www.csa.com>* . . . . *
- *Sociological Abstracts (SA) <www.csa.com>* 1992
- *Studies on Women Abstracts <www.tandf.co.uk>* 1982
- *SwetsNet <http://www.swetsnet.com>* 2002
- *Women Studies Abstracts* 1991
- *Women's Healthbeat* 1998
- *Women's Studies Index (indexed comprehensively)* 1992
- *World Agricultural Economics & Rural Sociology Abstracts*
  (c/o CAB Intl/CAB ACCESS) <www.cabi.org> 1992

*Exact start date to come.

(continued)

Special Bibliographic Notes related to special journal issues
(separates) and indexing/abstracting:

- indexing/abstracting services in this list will also cover material in any "separate" that is co-published simultaneously with Haworth's special thematic journal issue or DocuSerial. Indexing/abstracting usually covers material at the article/chapter level.
- monographic co-editions are intended for either non-subscribers or libraries which intend to purchase a second copy for their circulating collections.
- monographic co-editions are reported to all jobbers/wholesalers/approval plans. The source journal is listed as the "series" to assist the prevention of duplicate purchasing in the same manner utilized for books-in-series.
- to facilitate user/access services all indexing/abstracting services are encouraged to utilize the co-indexing entry note indicated at the bottom of the first page of each article/chapter/contribution.
- this is intended to assist a library user of any reference tool (whether print, electronic, online, or CD-ROM) to locate the monographic version if the library has purchased this version but not a subscription to the source journal.
- individual articles/chapters in any Haworth publication are also available through the Haworth Document Delivery Service (HDDS).

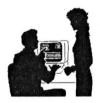

Teaching Gender, Teaching Women's Health: Case Studies in Medical and Health Science Education

CONTENTS

Teaching Gender, Teaching Women's Health: Introduction   1
Lenore Manderson, PhD, FASSA

Teaching Women's Health into the 21st Century   11
Naomi Rogers, PhD
Janet Henrich, MD

Exchanging Hats: A Gendered Perspective on Teaching
Clinical Medical Anthropology   23
Elizabeth Cartwright, PhD, RN

Gender in Medical Curricula: Course Organizer Views
of a Gender-Issues Perspective in Medicine in Sweden   35
Anna Westerståhl, MD, PhD
Maria Andersson, MD, PhD
Margareta Söderström, MD, PhD

Women Teaching Women's Health: Issues in the Establishment
of a Clinical Teaching Associate Program for the Well
Woman Check   49
Kathryn Robertson, MBBS, MEd
Kelsey Hegarty, MBBS, PhD
Vivienne O'Connor, MBChB
Jane Gunn, MBBS, PhD

Gender and the Medical Curriculum: A Rural Case Study   67
Jo Wainer, MA

Outing Lesbian Health in Medical Education   89
    Ruth McNair, MBBS, DRACOG, DA(UK), FRACGP,
    FACRRM

Not Only What You Do, But How You Do It: Working
    with Health Care Practitioners on Gender Equality   105
    Sharon Fonn, MBBCh, FFCH, PhD

The Integration of Gender in Medical Research and Education–
    Obstacles and Possibilities from a Nordic Perspective   121
    Anne Hammarström, MD, PhD

Index   135

ABOUT THE EDITOR

Lenore Manderson, PhD, is Professor of Women's Health at the Key Centre for Women's Health in Society for the University of Melbourne. A medical anthropologist known for her work in sociology, social history, and public health, she has conducted research on infectious and chronic disease, gender, and sexuality in Southeast and East Asia and Africa as well as Australia, in the latter case with immigrant and indigenous women and Anglo-Australians. In 2001, Professor Manderson was awarded an inaugural Federation Fellowship by the Australian Research Council, and she is conducting a five-year research program on chronic illness, disability, social relationships, and well-being. She is a Fellow of the Academy of Social Sciences in Australia and President of the International Association for the Study of Sexuality, Culture, and Society. Dr. Manderson has written several books, including *Australian Women's Health: Innovations in Social Science and Community Research, Sickness and the State: Health and Illness in Colonial Malaya, 1870-1940,* and *Sites of Desire/Economies of Pleasure* (with M. Jolly).

Teaching Gender,
Teaching Women's Health:
Introduction

Lenore Manderson, PhD, FASSA

There is an increasing, widespread awareness of the ways in which both biology and culture–sex and gender–affect the risks and prevalence of disease, and health outcomes, of men and women. In a recent issue of the *American Journal of Obstetrics & Gynecology*, for example, Phillips (2002) drew attention to the need for systematic teaching of gender, as an essential and integral component of medical training, and identified specific educational objectives along these lines. Others have made similar points of the need to incorporate sociological factors such as gender, and other variables such as age and class, in order to ensure appropriate care: Goldstein (2002) makes this same point with respect to the assessment and treatment of mental illness in primary care settings.

This awareness coincides with the increase in absolute numbers and proportion of women entering medical school. This trend is virtually worldwide, the result of general trends in gender equity, changes in secondary and pre-medical tertiary education, the encouragement of women into various fields of medicine previously dominated by men, and the demand by women patients for women general practitioners. By the mid 1980s, in countries such as the United States, the number of women enrolling at commencement of a medical

Lenore Manderson is affiliated with the Key Centre for Women's Health in Society, University of Melbourne, Victoria 3010, Australia (E-mail: lenorem@unimelb.edu.au).

[Haworth co-indexing entry note]: "Teaching Gender, Teaching Women's Health: Introduction." Manderson, Lenore. Co-published simultaneously in *Women & Health* (The Haworth Medical Press, an imprint of The Haworth Press, Inc.) Vol. 37, No. 4, 2003, pp. 1-9; and: *Teaching Gender, Teaching Women's Health: Case Studies in Medical and Health Science Education* (ed: Lenore Manderson) The Haworth Medical Press, an imprint of The Haworth Press, Inc., 2003, pp. 1-9. Single or multiple copies of this article are available for a fee from The Haworth Document Delivery Service [1-800-HAWORTH, 9:00 a.m. - 5:00 p.m. (EST). E-mail address: docdelivery@haworthpress.com].

degree was approaching that of men, although the proportion of women enrolled in all years was around 35 percent in most countries (Pizurki et al. 1987; Pringle 1998), indicating a greater attrition rate for women than men. US data also indicated an increasing proportion of women in residency training programs, in the number of practising physicians, and in female academic staff of medical schools (Braslow & Heins 1981; Bickel 1988; Levinson & Weiner 1991).

By the turn of the century, these trends appeared to have reached a plateau, with Bickel reporting in 2001 that women are still only 44% of enrollees. Similar patterns can be observed elsewhere, too; in Israel, for instance, the number of women who had graduated had increased by over 50% between 1981 and 1995, to 35.3% in the latter year, with a disproportionate number here as elsewhere choosing family medicine rather than specialist training and practice (Reis et al. 2001). Further, while it is not surprising for women to undertake medical training or to work as doctors, there are still specific factors that continue to discourage women from enrolling in and completing medical training, still disparities in women's versus men's careers (see further below), and still a number of ways in which gender influences the practice of medicine (Pringle 1998). Yet there has been limited scholarly attention to women's increased participation in the provision of medical care, and to the implications that this might have for medical training and practice.

This volume contributes to this literature across three broad fields. The first papers consider the ways in which gender issues are being introduced in pre-medical training and related health courses (Rogers and Henrich, and Cartwright), providing new data on the continuing challenges of introducing ideas of gender to in the classroom. The second set of papers explore innovations in medical education to enhance the quality of medical practice through the use of gender-issues perspective throughout the curricula (Westerståhl et al.), the use of lay teaching associates to train students to conduct gynecological examinations (Robertson et al.), and by encouraging women doctors to take up rural practice and to be aware of how gender factors influence the experiences of doctors and patients in rural environments (Wainer). A fourth paper in this set raises the need for a specific area of training, currently ignored in most medical curricula–this is the area of lesbian health (McNair). The third set of papers, by Fonn and Hammarström, consider the inclusion of gender from the respective points of view of primary health care trainers and researchers. None present particularly optimistic paths to the changes that the integration of gender foreshadows.

A number of researchers have recently noted that physicians bring to their training specific beliefs and values influenced by their own socialization, including with respect to sex and gender, and draw attention to the need for curricula changes (Phillips & Ferguson 1999; Weiss & Levinson 2000; Wong

2000). A study of undergraduate medical students in Canada, for instance, showed that while, as they matured, students were less accepting of gender stereotypes, they nevertheless maintained an implicit understanding of the male body as normative and conceptualized women as "other" or "abnormal" (Phillips & Ferguson 1999; see also Zelek et al. 1997 and cf. Beagan 2000). Others suggest that conventional stereotypical values marry with other professional values moulded in medical school (Coulehan & Williams 2001), often with important effects in terms of medical practice, specifically in terms of the treatment women experience as patients (Cox 1997). Integrating gender issues in medical education is therefore critical (Lent & Bishop 1998). However, where graduate entry to medical education is the norm, as is the case in the United States, there are earlier opportunities to introduce students to the concepts of sex and gender, and to how gender shapes health outcomes. The first papers in this volume describe educational innovations in this area.

In the first paper, Naomi Rogers and Janet Henrich describe the introduction, pedagogical approaches and responses to the Women's and Gender Studies Program provided at Yale University School of Medicine. The women's health course has now operated for almost a decade; it was introduced relatively early, inspired by feminist health politics of the 1970s, and it still unapologetically uses *Our Bodies, Our Selves* as a text. The course introduces undergraduate students to social and cultural aspects of women's health and gender, against a backdrop of what Rogers and Henrich portrays as "the shifting politics of women's health" in the United States. Elizabeth Cartwright describes her use of a gendered perspective in a clinical medical anthropology course at Idaho State University, in which she draws on material from the humanities as well as the social sciences to encourage students to think creatively about the social experiences of illness. Like the Yale course, this course too is innovative theoretically and pedagogically. In both papers, the authors include students' own reflections on the challenges to their taken-for-granted understandings of gender and social structure. Courses such as these are critical if we are to meet the needs of diverse populations of patients who are articulate in their expectations of their health providers and sensitive to shortfalls in their care.

Medical training requires students to develop a range of abilities both theoretic and technical. The reflective and analytic skills are those appropriate to the changing culture of medicine and nurtured in problem-based learning, where students must appreciate the ways in which economic, social and cultural factors, including gender, complicate patients' experiences of ill health and their presentation for care. For many students, such understanding comes hard. As those of us who have taught social science and public health are well aware, students are often impatient with what they perceive as "soft" science and "common-sense," far more interested in and concerned to master the principles of pathology, genetics and immunology and to gain the skills that they believe will directly translate into practice success. In medical school, it makes little sense to sequester gender-issues to obstetrics and gynecology, for example, and a gender-issues perspective assumes integration in all areas. However, there is not always support for this strategy. In this volume, Anna Westerståhl and colleagues describe the impact of a decision taken by the Medical Faculty of Göteborg University, Sweden, to include a gender-issues perspective in medical education. Three years on, course organizers from preclinical and clinical departments were interviewed to determine the extent to which they felt a gender-issues perspective was relevant to their field and if so, how this was incorporated into their teaching. Their data suggest that while women members of faculty felt the approach important and had ensured that their teaching reflected the changes in knowledge and understandings of gender in practice, male colleagues and students were skeptical or disinterested in the approach and saw little relevance of it to medical training and/or their own areas of expertise.

While there is little evidence that men and women emerge from their training with a different knowledge base, there does appear to be certain differences in styles of practice. Women are more likely than men to listen without interrupting, display empathy, allow patients time for discussion which may produce stronger rapport (Hojat et al. 2002a, 2002b), and to show more general attentiveness to the patient and perform longer and/or more complete physical examinations (van Dulmen & Bensing 2000; see also Carney et al. 2000). The differences that gender makes in practice have resulted in the strong preference of young women and minority women for female general practitioners (Bates & Linder-Pelz 1987: 51-53; Young et al. 1997; Kelaher et al. 1998; Kirk et al. 1998). This may be associated too with patient satisfaction and patient compliance with their therapeutic regimens (Arnold et al. 1988). However, the promotion of routine screening for cancer prevention appears to have had the major influence on women's preference for women providers. In Australia, where cervical cancer smears are undertaken by general practitioners, women doctors regularly remark on the disproportionate amount of time they spend on such procedures, while their male colleagues deal with the wider variety of health problems. In an attempt to improve the general quality of vaginal, breast and related examinations, thereby ensuring that all women will receive sensitive care regardless of the gender of their practitioner, Gynecology Teaching Associates have become increasingly routine in medical training in industrialized settings. Gynecology Teaching Associate programs, using specially trained standardized patients, were introduced in the USA from the late 1970s and are now routine in American and Canadian medical schools (Kretzschmar 1978); in Australia they have been introduced only in the past decade in a growing number of medical schools.

There are few published descriptions or evaluations of this approach in ensuring women's comfort with gynecological examination and the relationship of this to adherence to regular Pap smears (Kretzschmar 1978; Shain et al. 1982; Guenther et al. 1983), hence the importance of the paper by Kathryn Robertson and colleagues. These authors describe the Gynecology Teaching Associate programs of two medical schools at which this approach has been introduced in Australia, since 1996 at the University of Queensland, and from 2000 at the University of Melbourne. These programs aim to train medical students and doctors in the technical and communication skills to address women's general dissatisfaction and occasional distress in breast and gynecological examinations, and consequently, to encourage their participation in screening.

Women's concentration in general practice rather than into postgraduate specialist training is common, and relates in part to their perception of the incompatibility of specialist medicine and domestic roles. At least until a decade ago, postgraduate training was affected particularly by women's role in reproduction and the maintenance of family life, and women's patterns of enrolment in postgraduate medicine are consistent with the general low enrolment of women in higher degrees (Australian Tertiary Education Commission 1991). Research from the 1980s, although dated, provides clues to this: in the US and Australia following graduation, women are poorly represented in certain specialties, for reasons that include the lack of flexibility of post-graduate training and working, and the lack of compatibility of specialization with child-bearing, child-rearing and other domestic responsibilities. Yet at the same time, women tend to be overrepresented in other fields: in the US, in paediatrics, obstetrics and gynecology and pathology (for an early discussion, see Gordon 1989). In Australia, women are concentrated in the fields of anesthetics and psychiatry, and Redman et al. (1994) have argued the importance to women, in determining career choice, of flexible working hours, the possibility for combining work and other family-related activities, and part-time work. The disproportionately low numbers of women in specialties and their underrepresentation also in senior academic positions (Richman et al. 2001), means that there are few female role models or mentors to provide younger women with support, guidance and advice, and access to informal networks that facilitate career development (Bright et al. 1998).

Jo Wainer's paper, in relation to rural practice, describes how one medical school has recognized the importance of role models for women and included it in medical education, with the aim of encouraging women to work in an area of practice–rural general practice–that is famous for its difficulty in recruiting either men or women. Rural practice is at a particular disadvantage, given women's general propensity to take account of their partners' needs in making their own career choices, and their relative lack of mobility influencing location of employment and options for work following graduation. The teaching program described in Wainer's paper illustrates how one department sought to address both issues of gender and locality. At the same time as academic staff had to train tutors and meet students' needs by providing a framework within which to think about gender and medicine, it was necessary to work as advocates for the program with funding agencies, other faculty and students. As Wainer illustrates, the resistance to which Westerståhl and co-authors refer is not unique.

While through their choice of provider and consumer critiques, many women have drawn attention to the shortcomings of conventional medicine, lesbian consumers have been even more frustrated at the lack of sensitivity and knowledge that they experience in their interactions with providers, both men and women. As reflected in the report of the Institute of Medicine (IOM) (Solarz 1999), there is a growing awareness of the challenges of providing quality health care to lesbians, given continued evidence of homophobia and discriminatory behavior from health professionals, and expected or actual negative experiences in and lack of quality care (Bradford et al. 2001; Plumb 2001). Research with lesbians has concentrated on breast and cervical cancer, sexual and mental health, including alcohol abuse and violence. The Institute's report argues for a comprehensive research program but also points to the importance of addressing, through the training of health professionals and provision of services, barriers to good health among lesbians and other sexual minority women. In her contribution, Ruth McNair addresses the difficult task of introducing the field of lesbian health, a field excluded in most medical curricula. In this timely paper, McNair reviews how lesbian health is addressed in medical education programs, and argues for its inclusion in medical training.

This volume focuses on medical education, but health care is not the sole province of doctors, and many people in the world are more likely when ill to be assisted by other health providers. Sharon Fonn describes the innovative work of the Women's Health Project of the University of Witwatersrand, South Africa, which for the past decade has run a variety of gender and health training courses for health professionals, and has played a major role in the development of gender and reproductive health curricula. In this article, she describes the motivation behind and methods of the courses provided by the Project, in which adult learning techniques, small group discussions, role plays and other interactive methods are used to make concrete to course participants the importance of gender theory, the value of gender analysis, and the implications of this understanding to the everyday activities of the participants. She illustrates how structural and situational factors influence gender and health concerns for women, and discusses the impact of such training on participants and health services.

In general, participants of such courses complete their training with the confidence that they can make an impact on health policies and programs at their workplaces (Vlassoff & Fonn 2001), although more comprehensive change requires political will and commitment at all levels of government. Anne Hammarström provides a further example of the gaps between rhetoric and practice, drawing again on the experiences in the Nordic countries in integrating Gender in Medical Research and Education. Gender research has gained ground and respectability in Swedish medical faculties as a result of a strong political commitment for increased research and integration in teaching of gender issues in the university curriculum in Sweden. Within the academy, however, there has been considerable resistance, with some insisting on the irrelevance of gender to their fields of study and others seeking to narrow the scope to a more conventional characterization of obstetrics and gynecology. In research as in teaching, and in training, therefore, women have had to work as pioneers.

Biomedical and epidemiological research over the past decade has also drawn increased attention to the importance of gender in the presentation and course of disease, with implications in terms of treatment and prognosis. Social and cultural factors further influence outcomes, including women's access to care, choice of health provider, and the quality of care received. The increased attention paid to new knowledge and new perspectives has encouraged the incorporation of gender issues into medical curricula, not simply as an adjunct but as core to medical theory and practice. Yet, as a number of authors illustrate, noted above, changing practice and understanding is difficult even when there is formal commitment to gender-based medicine and analysis. In general, as Shelley and colleagues (2000) remark, health care policy and medical education has not taken on board the growing awareness of sex and gender differences. The case studies presented in this volume are pioneering work in this field, promising in the future better training and greater choices for women professionals, and better quality care for those who turn to them.

REFERENCES

Arnold, R.M., Martin, S.C. and R.M. Parker (1988). Taking care of patients: Does it matter whether the physician is a woman? *Western Journal of Medicine* 149: 729-733.

Australian Tertiary Education Commission (1991). *Selected Higher Education Statistics*. Belconnen, ACT: Australian Tertiary Education Commission.

Beagan, B.L. (2000). Neutralizing differences: producing neutral doctors for (almost) neutral patients. *Social Science and Medicine* 51 (8): 1253-1265.

Bickel, J. (1988). Women in medical education. A status report. *New England Journal of Medicine* 319 (24): 1579-1584.

Bickel, J. (2001). Gender equity in undergraduate medical education: a status report. *Journal of Womens Health & Gender-Based Medicine* 10 (3): 261-270.

Bradford, J., Ryan, C., Honnold, J. and E. Rothblum (2001). Expanding the research infrastructure for lesbian health. *American Journal of Public Health* 91(7): 1029-1032.

Braslow, J.B. and M. Heins (1981). Women in medical education: a decade of change. *New England Journal of Medicine* 304: 1129-1135.

Bright, C.M., Duefield, C.A. and V.E. Stone (1998). Perceived barriers and biases in the medical education experience by gender and race. *Journal of the National Medical Association* 90 (11): 681-688.

Carney, P.A., Dietrich, A.J., Eliassen, S., Pipas, C. and D. Donahue (2000). Differences in ambulatory teaching and learning by gender match of preceptors and students. *Family Medicine* 32 (9): 618-623.

Cartwright, L.K. (1972). Conscious factors entering into decisions of women to study medicine. *Journal of Social Issues* 28: 201-215.

Coulehan, J. and P.C. Williams (2001). Vanquishing virtue: the impact of medical education. *Academic Medicine* 76 (6): 598-605.

Cox, C. (1997). Medical education, women's status, and medical issues' effect on women's health in the Caribbean. *Health Care for Women International* 18 (4): 383-393.

Goldstein, M.Z. (2002). Depression and anxiety in older women. *Primary Care; Clinics in Office Practice* 29 (1): 69-80.

Gordon, J. (1989). Women in postgraduate training. *Australian Medicine* 1 (November 20): 423-430.

Guenther, S.M., Laube, D.W. and S. Matthes (1983). Effectiveness of the gynecology teaching associate in teaching pelvic examination skills. *Journal of Medical Education* 58 (1): 67-69.

Hojat, M., Gonnella, J.S., Nasca, T.J., Mangione, S., Vergare, M. and M. Magee (2002a). Physician empathy: definition, components, measurement, and relationship to gender and specialty. *American Journal of Psychiatry* 159 (9): 1563-1569.

Hojat, M., Gonnella, J.S., Mangione, S., Nasca, T.J., Veloski, J.J., Erdmann, J.B., Callahan, C.A. and M. Magee (2002b). Empathy in medical students as related to academic performance, clinical competence and gender. *Medical Education* 36 (6): 522-527.

Kelaher, M., Gillespie, A., Allotey, P., Manderson, L., Potts, H., Sheldrake, M. and M. Young (1998). *The Impact of Culture and Ethnicity on Cervical Screening in Queensland*. Report to Queensland Health. Brisbane: Queensland Health.

Kirk, M., Hoban, E., Dunne, A. and L. Manderson (1998). *Barriers to and Appropriate Delivery Systems for Cervical Cancer Screening in Indigenous Communities in Queensland: Final Report*. Brisbane: Queensland Health.

Kretzschmar, R.M. (1978). Evolution of the Gynecology Teaching Associate: an education specialist. *American Journal of Obstetrics & Gynecology* 131 (4): 367-373.

Lent, B. and J.E. Bishop (1998). Sense and sensitivity: developing a gender issues perspective in medical education. *Journal of Women's Health* 7 (3): 339-342.

Levinson, W. and J. Weiner (1991). Promotion and tenure of women and minorities on medical school faculties. *Annals of Internal Medicine* 114 (1): 63-68.

Phillips, S.P. (2002). Evaluating women's health and gender. *American Journal of Obstetrics and Gynecology* 187 (3 Supp): S22-24.

Phillips, S.P. and K.E. Ferguson (1999). Do students' attitudes toward women change during medical school? *CMAJ: Canadian Medical Association Journal* 160 (3): 357-361.

Pizurki, H., Mejia, A., Butler, I. and L. Ewart (1987). *Women as Providers of Health Care.* Geneva: World Health Organization.

Plumb, M. (2001). Undercounts and overstatements: will the IOM report on lesbian health improve research? *American Journal of Public Health* 91 (6): 873-875.

Pringle, R. (1998). *Sex and Medicine: Gender, Power and Authority in the Medical Profession.* Melbourne: Cambridge University Press.

Redman, S., Saltman, D., Straton, J., Young, B. and C. Paul (1994). Determinants of career choices among medical students and interns. *Medical Education* 28: 361-371.

Reis, S., Goldfracht, M., Tamir, A., van Raalte, R., Spenser, T. and D. Hermoni (2001). Trends in medical speciality choice among Israeli medical graduates, 1980-1995. *IMAJ: Israel Medical Association Journal* 3 (12): 973-977.

Richman, R.C., Morahan, P.S., Cohen, D.W. and S.A. McDade (2001). Advancing women and closing the leadership gap: The Executive Leadership in Academic Medicine (ELAM) program experience. *Journal of Women's Health & Gender-Based Medicine* 10 (3): 271-277.

Shain, R.N., Crouch, S.H. and P.C. Weinberg (1982). Evaluation of the gynecology teaching associate versus pelvic model approach to teaching pelvic examination. *Journal of Medical Education* 57 (8): 646-648.

Shelley, D., Hoffman, E., Menitoff, R. and P. Maraldo (2000). Quality in women's health. *Quality Management in Health Care* 8 (4): 65-74.

Solarz, A.L. (ed.) (1999). *Lesbian Health. Current Assessment and Directions for the Future.* Washington, DC: National Academy Press for Institute of Medicine.

van Dulmen, A.M. and J.M. Bensing (2000). Gender differences in gynecologist communication. *Women & Health* 30 (3): 49-61.

Vlassoff, C. and S. Fonn (2001). Health workers for change as a health systems management and development tool. *Health Policy & Planning* 16 (Supp. 1): 47-52.

Weiss, L.B. and S.P. Levinson (2000). Tools for integrating women's health into medical education: clinical cases and concept mapping. *Academic Medicine* 75 (11): 1081-1086.

Wong, Y.L. (2000). Gender issues in medical and pubic health education. *Asia-Pacific Journal of Public Health* 12 Supp.: S74-77.

Young, A.F., Byles, J.E. and A.J. Dobson (1998). Women's satisfaction with general practice consultations. *Medical Journal of Australia* 168: 386-389.

Zelek, B., Phillips, S.P. and Y. Lefebvre (1997). Gender sensitivity in medical curricula. *CMAJ: Canadian Medical Association Journal* 156 (9): 1297-1300.

Teaching Women's Health
into the 21st Century

Naomi Rogers, PhD
Janet Henrich, MD

SUMMARY. In this paper we explore the political background to the Women's Health course at Yale University, its structures and goals and some of its striking successes and failures. The Yale Women's Health course has been shaped by tensions between the generation of (mostly) women who teach the course and the distinctive expectations and interests of the women (and the few men) who are its students. Over the past decade, it has been part of the shifting politics of women's health in the United States. To be able to speculate about the future of undergraduate women's health teaching in this new century means confronting distinctive characteristics of the current generation of women and men. We explore some of these characteristics in this paper and examine how different lecture topics have engaged students. *[Article copies available for a fee from The Haworth Document Delivery Service: 1-800-HAWORTH. E-mail address: <docdelivery@haworthpress.com> Website: <http://www.HaworthPress. com> © 2003 by The Haworth Press, Inc. All rights reserved.]*

Naomi Rogers is Assistant Professor, Section of History of Medicine and Gender Studies Program, Yale University. Janet Henrich is Associate Professor of Medicine and Obstetrics and Gynecology, Yale University School of Medicine, Women's and Gender Studies Program.

Address correspondence to: Naomi Rogers, PhD, Section of History of Medicine, Yale University of Medicine, New Haven, CT 06510 USA (E-mail: naomi.rogers@ yale.edu).

[Haworth co-indexing entry note]: "Teaching Women's Health into the 21st Century." Rogers, Naomi, and Janet Henrich. Co-published simultaneously in *Women & Health* (The Haworth Medical Press, an imprint of The Haworth Press, Inc.) Vol. 37, No. 4, 2003, pp. 11-21; and: *Teaching Gender, Teaching Women's Health: Case Studies in Medical and Health Science Education* (ed: Lenore Manderson) The Haworth Medical Press, an imprint of The Haworth Press, Inc., 2003, pp. 11-21. Single or multiple copies of this article are available for a fee from The Haworth Document Delivery Service [1-800-HAWORTH, 9:00 a.m. - 5:00 p.m. (EST). E-mail address: docdelivery@haworthpress.com].

10.1300/J013v37n04_02

KEYWORDS. Women's health, gender and medicine, undergraduate teaching, health activism, women and research, women's health politics

Students taking the Yale University undergraduate course Women's Health must write a 10-12 page research paper on a topic of their own choosing, some of which are listed below. For most students this project is the most satisfying part of the course. Depression, eating disorders, contraception and female genital mutilation are consistently popular subjects, as are ones that have special meaning for the writer. The papers are intended as reviews of the scientific and/or social science literature, but many students also include personal stories or experiences on a family member.

- female orgasm during intercourse: a joint effort
- prosecution of crack mothers: a crisis of morality or public health?
- the ordinary and the beautiful: cosmetic surgery and minority women
- comparison of egg and sperm donation .
- why society encourages women to deny their age
- eating disorders in female athletes
- menstruation in the history of China

The evolution of Yale's Women's Health course over the past decade is part of the shifting politics of women's health in the United States.[1] It has been and continues to be shaped by tensions between the generation of (mostly) women who teach the course and the distinctive expectations and interests of the women (and a few men) who are its students. In this paper we explore the political and institutional background to the course, its structure and goals, and some of its striking successes and failures. Speculating about the future of undergraduate women's health teaching in this new century means confronting the distinctive characteristics of a generation of young women and men who were born after HIV/AIDS was identified and became a normalized part of daily news reports; became sexually active after the peak years of the sexual revolution, the feminist health movement, and the gay rights movement; entered tertiary institutions that had institutionalized (however marginally) women's studies courses, journals, and the other trappings of academe; and face a world where the presence of prominent women in politics, sport and science is taken for granted, and popular magazines and television talk shows feature breast cancer, childhood sexual abuse, eating disorders, and the transgendered.[2]

First offered in 1994, the Women's Health course was designed and run by two Yale Medical School faculty members: internist Janet B. Henrich, Associate Professor of Medicine and Obstetrics/Gynecology and psychologist Linda M. Bartoshuk, Professor of Surgery and Psychology. Both were experienced in women's health politics in Washington, DC, and wanted to inspire younger women to consider careers in the burgeoning field of women's health. Their departments somewhat reluctantly agreed that they could take (unpaid) time to teach this new course.

The early 1990s was a time of dramatic change in the funding and visibility of women's health policy and biomedical research. A growing awareness of the biomedical community's neglect of research into women's health problems and the need to provide women with equal access to the benefits of such research was spurred by public outrage over the so-called Aspirin Study (Physicians' Health Study), whose publicized report in 1989 on the efficacy of aspirin in preventing heart disease was based on a study of some 22 thousand male physicians–and not one woman.[3] The Congressional Caucus for Women's Issues (set up in 1977 to try to implement the Equal Rights Amendment) and other state and federal politicians recognized the political urgency of these issues, as many government lobbyists, consumer advocates and politicians were facing breast cancer, ovarian cancer or post-menopausal depression themselves or in members of their families. This political and public pressure led to a widely-publicized government report by the General Accounting Office in 1990, showing that the federal National Institutes of Health (NIH)'s own guidelines for the representation and integration of women as subjects of research were not being followed or enforced. In 1990 NIH issued new, more stringent guidelines, and also established an Office of Research on Women's Health. In 1991, cardiologist Bernadine Healy was appointed as the NIH's first-ever woman director. At a conference in Hunt Valley, Maryland, convened by Healy to bring together women's health experts from government, the biomedical community and health advocacy groups across North America, speakers in talk after talk detailed the ways women were excluded or under-represented as subjects in federally-funded research.[4] Healy announced the funding of the Women's Health Initiative which she called a "moonwalk for women," the first massive (14 year, $625 million) government-supported clinical trial organized around the health problems of older women (aged 50-79) and largely directed and staffed by women (as researchers, clinicians, and patients). Congress provided significant federal funding for breast cancer research, and set up women's health centers at the Veterans Administration. Other federal health agencies like the Centers for Disease Control and the Food and Drug Administration established their own women's health offices, and the Public Health Service began funding Centers of Excellence in Women's Health at academic medical centers across the country, intended to promote a new model of health care for women, through the integration and transformation of clinical practice, education and research. The ambitious goals of these Centers–14 by 2001–included: promoting women professionals at academic health centers, attracting younger researchers into women's health research, and working with consumer and advocacy groups to develop public education in women's health.[5] A few university teaching programs were also developed. In 1990 the University of Illinois at Chicago's graduate nursing program offered a course in women's health, and similar gender and health graduate courses were begun at the University of Maryland and through the Women's Studies Center at the University of Florida. Women's studies faculty at the University of Wisconsin at Madison had been teaching a women's health course since the early 1980s.[6]

Yale was one of many universities to draw on these resources. A leading center for medical research and teaching in North America, Yale was one of six sites first selected to become a Center of Excellence in Women's Health. Gynecologist-researcher Florence Haseltine was an early regular lecturer in the Women's Health course, presenting students with her provocative personal perspectives as one of the NIH researchers who had set up the Society for the Advancement of Women's Health Research and its journal, *Journal of Women's Health and Gender-Based Medicine*, part of a growing number of refereed women's health science journals.[7] Hospitals and universities around the United States began to recognize a burgeoning women's health market, and in October 1992 there was the politically astute publication of a special issue on women's health by the *Journal of the American Medical Association (JAMA)*. In March 2001 *JAMA*, under its first-ever woman editor, repeated the experiment, and received over 200 manuscript submissions.[8] The Yale course reader (a collection of articles and extracts updated every two years) relies on these publications, such as *Women and Health, Gender and Society, Women's Health Issues, Journal of Women's Health*, as well as the more mainstream *JAMA, American Journal of Public Health, New England Journal of Medicine*, and the medicine and science reporting of the *New York Times*.

The women's health lecture course first offered in spring term 1994 was almost a disaster, due to its own tremendous success. 178 students enrolled–an extraordinary number at a university that runs seminars for only 5 or 6 people, and considers lecture courses large if they attract over 50 students. Henrich and Bartoshuk were completely unprepared for the high turnout and for the responsibilities of reading and marking so many student papers. Further, they were chagrined to find that a number of their friends and colleagues who had agreed to give guest lectures were uncomfortable talking to a room full of undergraduates quick to sense condescension and to reject what they considered patronizing and boring simplification.

In 1995 Naomi Rogers, a historian of medicine, trained as an academic lecturer as well as researcher, began to help coordinate the course and turn it into a well-run, more typical Yale undergraduate lecture course, continuing its commitment to interdisciplinary and diverse perspectives on a variety of women's health topics. This structure remains the strength of the course today. She put together a more accessible reading packet and introduced weekly discussion sessions, so that students had a structured opportunity to respond to the readings and lectures. Enrolment was capped at 100. Since then the course has been offered every spring term, attracting around 60-80 students.

The semester-long course is open to Yale undergraduates at all levels, without prerequisites. Its formal requirements are: a one-hour midterm exam (20% of final grade), a 10-12 page research paper (45%), a three-hour final exam (25%), and class participation in discussion section (10%). The students, ranging in age from 17 to 22, are predominantly female, although a small number of male students enrol each year. The majority of students are interested in pursuing careers in the biomedical sciences or in public health and health policy; others have interests in law, journalism, the environment, and the creative and performing arts. As Yale's medical school does not teach undergraduates, the course is run under the auspices of the Women's and Gender Studies Program in the Faculty of Arts and Sciences. The course is run on a minimal budget, no speaker is paid, and there is almost no travel money (occasionally a train ticket for a New York speaker, paid from the modest Women's Studies budget). We rely on the university's rather aged audio-visual equipment; the science and clinical faculty have learned to bring their own laser pointers. There are 2 lectures a week and weekly discussion sections or tutorials led by graduate student teaching assistants drawn from around the university from such fields as Nurse-Midwifery, Psychology, Anthropology, Genetics, Epidemiology and Public Health, Forestry and Comparative Literature.

The lecturers–some 20 or so in a 14-week term–are an unusual combination of medical school clinicians, science and social science faculty, and community activists. They discuss areas of women's health that are at the heart of their own research or practice; some focus on the clinical aspects of a topic, others the psycho-social or political-ethical. All seek to supplement knowledge students have gained from family, peers and popular media, to challenge any simplistic or mistaken notions from these sources, and to offer useful, accessible and provocative information and ways of thinking about health across disciplines.

Lecturers have included a psychologist who heads Yale's eating disorders clinic; a physician who set up and ran Yale's women and AIDS primary care clinic; researcher-clinicians from Yale's substance abuse center and its STD clinic; a psychologist-researcher who specializes in women and depression; and a health ethics lawyer who taught "physician responsibility" (a compulsory course) to Yale's medical students. A sociologist who organizes a social science policy group on AIDS explains her ethnographic study of New Haven sex workers who are HIV positive; an epidemiologist from Yale's Department of Epidemiology and Public Health asks students to design a study investigating occupational disease among women employees of dry-cleaning stores; and the head of Yale's Department of Genetics reflects on the clinical and ethical implications of the pre-natal diagnostic testing his department provides. These speakers also provide advice to students exploring research topics, and sometimes clinicians and laboratory researchers offer them summer internships. "My reward for lecturing in the course," one professor told us, "is that I have the opportunity to recruit the best students as research assistants." After graduating, one of our students became a summer intern at the NIH's Office of Research on Women's Health; another got a job as a researcher for television music video station MTV's health program for teenagers, Mega-Dose.

The lectures that have been our most spectacular successes have much to do with the people who present them. Topics that constantly pull crowds are on women and domestic violence, breast cancer, women and depression, eating disorders, and egg donation. Some of the most memorable lectures have featured patients, a teaching method unfamiliar to most undergraduates. A clinician speaking on women and substance abuse gave some overview points, and then introduced a patient from his clinic, a nervous African-American woman who soon had students spell-bound with her story and her frank self-awareness. A medical internist, a recent graduate from Yale's medical school, discussed domestic violence, and brought one of her patients, a survivor not much older than our students, whose reflections left the student audience horrified, moved, and eager to talk.

The course is profoundly restricted by a lack of money and limited resources, even at this major research institution. We have, for example, rarely been able to find local researchers pursuing topics like women in the developing world, international health issues, or reproductive health. Further, the course line-up is consistently buffeted by speakers going on leave, leaving the university, getting tenure and at times refusing to continue participating (having done their civic time), and by shifting political coalitions within the medical school.

The course's goals have broadened since its inception, from inspiring young women to consider women's health as a serious career option to a kind of public education in women's health issues, but with a critical and intellectual edge, not as a substitute for reading popular magazines like *Cosmopolitan*. Speakers and students continue to provide enormous energy and enthusiasm, which makes it an enjoyable course to teach and direct. Student evaluations frequently say, "the best course I've had at Yale" and "every Yale woman should take it." Women students have told their boyfriends and male friends to enrol. During and especially in the discussion time near the end of lectures, students quiz speakers with little deference: they pressed a psychiatrist talking about women and mental health to say more about insurance coverage and the problems of elderly women whose depression was taken for granted.

The feminist health text *Our Bodies, Ourselves* is required,–and becomes a kind of litmus test for students.[9] Some see it as a crucial resource that will also be part of their personal library; others consider its politicized message offensive and a sign that this course attacks physicians and orthodox medicine (even though the current edition offers a much diluted version of the political power of the first 1971 edition). We continue to use feminist teaching materials and confront our post-feminist students, whose anonymous written comments as part of the course's final week assessment have included the enthusiastic:

- good to learn about your own body; what may face you in the future, and how to start to effect change to solve some of the problems that women suffer (1998)
- essential for women AND men. The personalized perspectives on an entire range of pertinent subjects makes the class a fascinating and informative and personally relevant experience (2000)

and the negative:

- it is ridiculous to ignore or marginalize modern medicine, this course should be renamed Women's Feelings and Issues because that is what it is about, not about women's health (2000)
- as a pre-med I am saddened that many lectures are anti-doctors . . . This should be changed (2000)
- I found 90% of the lectures to be either blatant distortions of reality (and attempts at indoctrinating impressionable young women) or even borderline offensive. This course had a myopic, and not terribly realistic, view of how issues of women's health should be approached (2000)

Students are suspicious that this course is a politicized effort to inculcate feminist views into the scientific world. Many of our lecturers, perhaps consciously, tend to dress formally and conservatively, and only one speaker, a local health educator talking about female sexuality, has ever looked remotely hippie-ish. Indeed, the course's most spectacular failures have had to do in part from this suspicion of old-style feminism and from the ages of the students. No speaker has been able to tread the delicate balance required in discussing female sexuality and reproductive health and disease between information (to a crowd that considers it knows everything, sort of) and education. A prominent sexology educator was considered too basic; an engaging gynecologist skilled in teenage girl's health and sexuality education was considered patronizing. An older sex therapist who looked like everyone's grandmother discussed her transgendered patients, but confronting the notion of people wanting to alter their sexual identities made young people still coming to terms with their own identities uneasy and unsympathetic.

Students have also rejected women's health activists. The executive director of the local Planned Parenthood organization who talked about abortion was considered unbalanced (and students asked us why we didn't also invite in a representative from anti-abortion groups). Barbara Seaman, the eminent feminist health advocate, was excited to come and talk to Yale women under-graduates, but her passionate discussion of the dangers of hormonal contraception alienated and annoyed the students. An organizer of a regional lesbian and gay health clinic spoke frankly and movingly about going to an emergency room with her lover and being rejected as not part of the immediate family, and of being told by her physician that her disinterest in learning about birth control was dangerous and irresponsible. Students did not find the lecture engaging or intellectually challenging. In 2001 we decided to introduce the topic of intersex, and, unable to find any local researchers, Rogers lectured herself and then showed a video produced by the Intersex Society of North America (ISNA). The video was provocative and effective, but later some students complained that they wanted to hear the "other point of view."

A change that was difficult for the course's original organizers to recognize was the shifting context between the mid-90s when women's health research entering into national science policy was new and exciting, and the late 1990s when students found three or four lectures on women's health research and policy redundant, and stories of the making of the Women's Health Initiative and ensuring the integration of women and minority subjects into NIH policy interesting only in a historical way. Our task was, thus, to shorten the course's initial pride in featuring many of the field's founding mothers. We have now only one left, and her lecture is listened to as one would hear the story of a woman who helped get the vote for women or force the Supreme Court to rule that sending birth control devices through the mail was not obscene–old feminist history, in other words.

SOME REFLECTIONS

As women's health educators who seek to engage young women look into the 21st century, we see that women's health is increasingly conceived as a legitimate field of inquiry. The idea of a women's health speciality is less frequently raised, but Yale, like other academic health centers, has adapted what Judith Lorber has called "strategy of wide-ranging woman-centered medicine."[10] Women's health has become a profitable and visible commodity in the health care and academic marketplaces.

The focus of women's health activism and policy making, however, has tended over the past few years to be on topics of greatest interest to older women. A local chapter of the National Organization for Women planning a conference on women's health called Yale last year to ask advice: their members wanted to attract younger women and so were thinking about having a session on breast cancer. We gently suggested a few other areas. Popular magazines oriented to young women continue to provide copious health sections, but other forums are less consistent. The health program Mega-Dose on MTV, directed to young women, for example, is no longer on. In 2000 the Eighth Annual Congress on Women's Health and Gender-Based Medicine had as its featured speaker Jane Fonda. Researchers in this field now have a shared community and their work speaks most often to the problems of mid-career professionals. The Ninth Annual Congress on Women's Health and Gender-Based Medicine, held in 2001, for example, had sessions on how to lobby on Capitol Hill for women's health research, how to set up a women's health center at your hospital, and where to find funding for women's health projects. The generation gap was clear in sessions such as: The Health of Our Daughters: Growing Up Faster Than Ever, Is Hooking Up Having Sex: What Our Daughters Are Up To and, in sessions brought back by popular demand, Lifestyle Management for the Female Physician, Dr. and Dr.: Dual Physician Marriages, and Stress and the Woman Physician: Dealing with the Overload Factor. The *Journal of Women's Health and Gender-Based Medicine* had a recent thematic issue on aging and sexuality, and in 2001 the journal *Women's Health Issues* explored mammography-related anxiety, and how to plan a successful women's health and wellness conference.

It is encouraging to see that many women's health leaders are now part of the medical and policy establishments. The women can and do act as role models and mentors. But the task of reaching and engaging the next generation of researchers, consumers and clients remains crucial. As the experience of directing Yale's undergraduate Women's Health course suggests, there are cultural, pedagogic and structural pitfalls that must be recognized and avoided. But we have taught no other course where our students tell us that it "changed their lives"–and mean it.

NOTES

1. For useful overviews see Susan Sherwin et al., eds. (1998) *The Politics of Women's Health: Exploring Agency and Autonomy*, Philadelphia: Temple University Press. Judith Walzer Leavitt, ed. (1999) *Women and Health in America: Historical Readings 2nd edition*, Madison: University of Wisconsin Press. Sheryl Burt Ruzek (1978) *The Women's Health Movement: Feminist Alternatives to Medical Control*, New York: Praeger. Barbara Bair and Susan E. Cayleff, eds. (1993) *Wings of Gauze: Women of Color and the Experience of Health and Illness,* Detroit: Wayne State University Press.

2. For historical and contemporary examples see Gary Null and Barbara Seaman (1999) *For Women Only: Your Guide to Health Empowerment*, New York: Seven Stories Press.

3. See for example JoDean Nicolette (2000) Searching for Women's Health: A Resident's Perspective, *Journal of Women's Health and Gender-Based Medicine*, 9, 697-701.

4. See for example Carol Sachs Weisman (1999) *Women's Health Care: Activist Traditions and Institutional Change*, Baltimore: Johns Hopkins University Press, 78-80. Elizabeth Fee and Nancy Krieger, eds. (1994) *Women's Health, Politics, and Power: Essays on Sex/Gender, Medicine, and Public Health*, Amityville, NY: Baywood.

5. Carol S. Weisman and Gayle L. Squires (2000) Women's Health Centers: Are the National Centers of Excellence in Women's Health a New Model? *Women's Health Issues*, 10, 248-255. Valeria M. Gwinner, Jerome F. Strauss, Nancy Miliken and Glenda D. Donoghue (2000) Implementing a New Model of Integrated Women's Health in Academic Health Centers: Lessons Learned from the National Centers of Excellence in Women's Health, *Journal of Women's Health & Gender-Based Medicine*, 9, 979-985. Carolyn M. Mazure, Mark Espeland, Pamela Douglas, Victoria Champion, and Marcia Killien (2000) Multidisciplinary Women's Health Research: The National Centers of Excellence in Women's Health, *Journal of Women's Health & Gender-Based Medicine*, 9, 717-722. Janet Bickel (2000) Women in Academic Medicine, *JAMA*, 55, 10-12.

6. For some overviews of this period see: Weisman (1999) *Women's Health Care*; and Nancy Worcester & Marianne H. Whatley, eds. (1994) *Women's Health: Readings on Social, Economic, and Political Issues* 2nd ed. Dubuque, Iowa: Kendall/Hunt; and on medical school teaching see Anna Day (1998) Teaching Women's Health: The Postgraduate Curriculum in Internal Medicine, *Annals RCPSC*, 31, 279-281.

7. Florence B. Haseltine and Beverly Jacobson, eds. (1997) *Women's Health Research: A Medical and Policy Primer*, Washington, DC: Health Press International.

8. Catherine D. De Angelis and Margaret A. Winker (2000) Women's Health: Filling the Gaps, *JAMA*, 285, 1508-1509. De Angelis and Winker (2000) Women's Health: A Call for Papers, *JAMA*, 283, 2714.

9. Boston Women's Health Book Collective (1998) *Our Bodies, Ourselves for the New Century*, New York: Simon and Schuster.

10. Judith Lorber A. (2000) What Impact Have Women Physicians Had on Women's Health? *JAMWA*, 55, 14.

APPENDIX

EXTRACTS FROM MIDTERM AND FINAL EXAMS, WGST 353B WOMEN'S HEALTH, YALE UNIVERSITY

You have just been chosen as special assistant to the Director of the National Institutes of Health. Your first assignment is to develop a research agenda for women's health as we head into the next millennium. Identify your three (3) highest priority areas of research and provide a rationale for each. Be sure to cite current and historical developments. (midterm 1995)

You are an occupational health researcher. Video Display Terminal (VDT) operators are complaining that they seem to have a high rate of miscarriage. How will you examine the validity of their claims? Describe 2 possible study designs and discuss the factors that will make them difficult to pursue. (midterm 1996)

What are the political and medical controversies around the issue of fetal health in relation to women's health? How do science and policy interact with respect to this issue? (midterm 1996)

Why is the fact that heart disease is the major cause of death in women the best kept secret in medicine? (midterm 1997)

Women have been consistently excluded from health research and medical product development. Does this exclusion justify the recent politicized attention to particular issues, such as breast cancer? Is political pressure a good way to allocate funds? (final 1997)

In what ways is HIV/AIDS a women's health issue? Discuss, with reference to socioeconomic and clinical aspects. (midterm 1998)

Design a syllabus for a Women's Health course. You must:

1. provide an organization theme for your course.

    • Justify how topics relate to each other and why you have chosen each lecture for the course.

2. include:

    • five lectures, each with a title
    • two assigned readings for each lecture
    • a paragraph describing your reasoning for this particular lecture's presence in the course. (final 2000)

Exchanging Hats:
A Gendered Perspective
on Teaching Clinical Medical Anthropology

Elizabeth Cartwright, PhD, RN

SUMMARY. This article outlines the progression of topics used to highlight gender in a clinical medical anthropology class. As the class moves through themes such as the use of high-technology medicine and doctor-patient communication, issues of the socially constructed nature of gender are brought to the fore. Included in this article are students' reflections on how they try to make sense of diverse notions of human sex-

Elizabeth Cartwright is Assistant Professor, Department of Anthropology, Idaho State University, where she teaches courses in medical and clinical anthropology, international health, and ethnographic methods. She is adjunct faculty in medical anthropology at *El Colegio de Sonora* (Hermosillo, Mexico). Dr. Cartwright serves as Director of the Binational Anthropology Field School (Idaho State) in Guanajuato, Mexico and of the Hispanic Health Projects, a bi-national team of researchers in studies on medical and social problems of Mexican farmworkers in Idaho. She has conducted clinical medical anthropology studies both in the US and in Latin America and has published widely on women's and children's health issues.

Address correspondence to: Elizabeth Cartwright, Department of Anthropology, Idaho State University, Pocatello, ID 83209 USA (E-mail: carteliz@isu.edu).

The author would like to thank the students who participated in the Clinical Medical Anthropology Seminar, Fall 2001. The discussions in that class resulted, in large part, in this article. It is students like these that make teaching a joy: Heather Schaper, Terry Livingston, Brian Mangum, Diana Campanella, Devon Denny, Shannon Case, Sheri Murphy, Rachel Carlson, and Rebecca Roberts.

[Haworth co-indexing entry note]: "Exchanging Hats: A Gendered Perspective on Teaching Clinical Medical Anthropology." Cartwright, Elizabeth. Co-published simultaneously in *Women & Health* (The Haworth Medical Press, an imprint of The Haworth Press, Inc.) Vol. 37, No. 4, 2003, pp. 23-34; and: *Teaching Gender, Teaching Women's Health: Case Studies in Medical and Health Science Education* (ed: Lenore Manderson) The Haworth Medical Press, an imprint of The Haworth Press, Inc., 2003, pp. 23-34. Single or multiple copies of this article are available for a fee from The Haworth Document Delivery Service [1-800-HAWORTH, 9:00 a.m. - 5:00 p.m. (EST). E-mail address: docdelivery@haworthpress.com].

10.1300/J013v37n04_03

uality and gender identity, and how these insights can be included in anthropological studies of clinical spaces. *[Article copies available for a fee from The Haworth Document Delivery Service: 1-800-HAWORTH. E-mail address: <docdelivery@haworthpress.com> Website: <http://www.HaworthPress.com> © 2003 by The Haworth Press, Inc. All rights reserved.]*

KEYWORDS. Clinical medical anthropology, gender, pedagogy

Unfunny uncles who insist
In trying on a lady's hat,
–oh, even if the joke falls flat,
we share your slight transvestite twist.

In spite of our embarrassment.
Costume and custom are complex.
The headgear of the other sex
Inspires us to experiment.

Elizabeth Bishop, 1956

This article explores the way in which gender can be given intellectual relief against the backdrop of a class in clinical medical anthropology. Through the use of ethnographies of the clinical spaces that make up the world of high-tech biomedicine, students are introduced into alternate realities where moral authority is enacted out through sacrosanct medical protocols. Using the concept to challenge the inscribed moral order and authority of the biomedical institution, students are led through a critical reasoning process. Ethnography, fiction, poetry and medical textbooks are all analyzed. This class is targeted to a multidisciplinary group of senior undergraduates and masters students of the social and clinical sciences.

The students work through the texts, analyzing them both for content and differences with respect to gender, ethnicity and socio-economic status. While highlighting gender in this discussion, ethnicity and socio-economic status are also integral axes of analysis. The class first moves through a discussion of illness narratives and conversation analysis of doctor-patient communication. We then address the theoretical issues of stigmatization and the cultural construction of risk–emphasizing how gender contributes to both of these processes. Expanding out from the focus on the patient, we begin to examine the clinical reality of medical doctors, questioning how clinicians are trained and the ramifications of the training regimen on how they ultimately work with their patients. Ethnographies and social analysis of birthing are used to highlight the culturally constructed nature of biological events–events that could be seen as "normal" and "healthy" or as "abnormal" and "pathological," depending on the perspective of the beholder. The last section of the class deals with specific illnesses such as AIDS and cancer, highlighting disparities in the illness trajectory from genetic testing, to scenarios of diagnosis and treatment, to dealing with the eventual outcome of death.

I include transcripts of class discussions and excerpts of students' written works in order to show the multiple interpretations of the literature. While teaching this class during the Fall of 2001, I enlisted the participation of the students in contributing to this article. Several of the class sessions were tape-recorded and segments of those transcriptions as well as short excerpts from weekly written memos are included in the following discussion of teaching gender.

BEGINNING WITH THEIR STORIES

Patients' stories provide an excellent entré into exploring the meaning of clinical spaces. Illness stories have the power to engage and illustrate how we construct our selves differently, in different social situations. Patients and clinicians alike tell stories of illnesses and clinical encounters in order to make meaning out of difficult events (Becker 1997). These stories are told again and again in order to establish not so much what "really" happened, but what sense we can make of it (LeGuin 1981, Polanyi 1981). Illness narratives are constructed to emphasize who was right and who was wrong (Price 1987). They point out blame for what can be interpreted retrospectively as clinical errors, misjudgements and outright mistakes, and they are deeply reflective of the local cultural moral order. By beginning with clinical narratives, the alternate logic of clinical spaces can begin to emerge as the background for the semester's class discussions.

Anthropology highlights local logics. Seen from outside, the progression of events in hospitals and clinics often appears to be arbitrary and capricious. Taking an emic or insider's point of view, clinical medical anthropologists try to see why these institutions function as they do. As anthropologists, using the emic point of view, we question why the "naturalized" social order exists as it does. To question this can be threatening for students. The pedagical question becomes, how do we get our students to try on these different spectacles, these different hats, especially when they fear how they might make the world look or feel?

> I'm sitting in a cardiologist's waiting room filling out my intake forms. The tip of my pen hovers above the ubiquitous binary boxes. Female or Male? I was born female-bodied and I identify as female–as a lesbian butch. However, some people see me as a feminine male. And whether they guess male or female, I am always perceived as "queer" because my

gender expression is very fluid and complex. I am transgender. Which box do I check to get the medical attention I need so badly right now? (Feinberg 2001:897)

I expect that it is when we catch the students just a touch off-guard that we make the most difference. We tuck something in that challenges preconceived ideas and allows students space to listen and to glimpse what being in another way might really be like. But we do this with the urgency of things clinical. It is the patient in the waiting room, with the difficult-to-diagnose disease or the raging infection, who needs help now. The clinical frenzy that surrounds urgent care clinics and emergency rooms generates enough adrenaline to get practitioners through the day; its addictive qualities make sure that they'll be back for another shift in the morning. That infective energy also can drive the compassion that we want to tap for our students.

Most good cultural anthropology conducted in clinical settings includes some sort of participant-observation or ethnographic description. The best of these ethnographic writings give us the imaginative distance needed to begin to see patterns of practice and interaction and to question the hegemonic institution of biomedicine.

Starting with the mysteries of birth, this class moves through the clinical maze of curing bodies both culturally wrought and institutionally controlled (Foucault 1973, Davis-Floyd 1992, Devries et al. 2001). Highlighting the cultural construction of the physiological process of birth demonstrates how women and their bodies articulate with institutions, how they are defined as normal or abnormal, and whether they are allowed more or less control over their birthing experiences. The notion that the physical process of birth can be defined as a medical event or a natural process lies at the root of a gendered reading of the medical system. It decenters the biomedically given reality that defines what is dangerous, wild, and in need of control. It also challenges what we take for granted as the "biomedical truth."

If we can challenge the notion that healthy women belong in institutions when they are birthing, then all the events surrounding a normal birth in an institution become cultural artifacts reflective of deeply held societal values. The cultural events that either put or do not put a birthing woman under the control of a biomedical practitioner are rich in analytical potential with respect to gender power hierarchies in the clinic and in the wider societal context (e.g., DeVries et al. 2001).

CONVERSATION ANALYSIS IN THE CLINICAL SETTING

In order to take apart the then-apparently culturally constructed power hierarchies, we turn to an analysis of doctor-patient communication. Using works that include transcripts of actual practitioner-patient conversations, the class examines how the world of biomedicine and the lifeworld of the patient are often very different and how that difference makes even the most simple exchange of information quite difficult at times (Habermas 1984, Mishler 1984, Barry et al. 2001). How do doctors talk to patients? Who is in control of the information? Who gets to express their point of view?

Based on the early works of Sacks, Schegeloff and Jefferson (1974), the analysis of turns at talk in the clinical encounter precisely describes what goes on when doctors talk to patients. Who has the conversational floor? How are turns at talk manipulated to the advantage of the doctor or the patient? How are encounters influenced by others present and by cultural expectations of verbal exchanges (Moerman 1988)? Once understood as a tool that clarifies power relationships, conversation analysis of medical encounters can be applied to a focused critique of gender specific issues within medical institutions (Fisher and Todd 1983). A multitude of questions comes from critiquing clinical conversations in this manner. Are birthing women really given choices or are their clinical encounters structured in a way that prevents them from having the information to question the biomedical system in the first place? Are these women physically moved through hospitals and clinics at a pace and in an atmosphere that precludes their equal participation in even basic discussions with medical personnel (Hopkins 2000)? By highlighting what happens when patients are placed in the position of making decisions when they are in pain or when they do not have adequate information, the power hierarchies inherent in the medical system become apparent. Often, this leads to a class discussion and critique of the concept of "informed consent."

THE CULTURAL CONSTRUCTION OF RISK AND STIGMATIZED POPULATIONS

In hospitals and clinics in many countries, as soon as clinicians and their patients begin discussing informed consents, the topic of risk comes up. Anthropologists argue that the concept of "risk" is a cultural construct (Douglas 1992). What is seen as risky in one society or culture may well not be seen as risky within another. The concept of risk includes what is locally accepted to be dangerous and it includes the idea that the possibility that one will personally be confronted with that danger can be mathematically determined (Skolbekken 1995).

The role of the anthropologist in analyzing risk is to focus on the process of cultural choice when it comes to what we are afraid of. Why are we afraid of home births and not the iatrogenic problems that come from giving birth in the hospital? How do the locally available medical technologies and the particular medico-legal system affect what patients and practitioners are afraid of (Cartwright and Thomas 2001)? Practitioners are often forced into practicing defensively to avoid malpractice lawsuits. Defensive medicine goes hand in hand with clinicians trying to exert more control over patients. Those who lose in this equation may well be those that are at a gender disadvantage.

Beyond being an exclusively "feminist" or "gay" issue, the continuum of human sexuality presents myriad problematic situations within the clinical setting that may affect a patient's access to appropriate and sensitive medical treatment. A more comprehensive and perhaps less limiting view of the expression of one's sexual identity and the range of possible forms of sexual attraction would include understanding standard feminist critiques and men's responses to those as well as lesbian, gay, bisexual and transgender perspectives (LGBT). A recent issue of the *American Journal of Public Health* addressed "LGBT" issues (the first time in its 91 year history as the author of one of these articles points out) with the following caveat:

> There are various gay male, lesbian, bisexual, and transgender populations: urban and rural, White and Black, poor and wealthy, and so forth. We refer to all of these as LGBT communities, but in doing so we risk glossing over important differences. White gay men in New York City's Chelsea neighborhood share little with transgender sex workers just a few blocks away in Grennwich Village; with gay men developing a gay liberation movement in Guadalajara, Mexico, with lesbians in Northhampton, Mass. or with bisexual married women on Long Island, NY. (Meyer 2001:854)

> In my medical classes (to be transgender) is presented as more of a rare condition and not a human thing . . . this is the freak of nature, this is what happens when the chromosomes are messed up, and not an everyday issue. The way that she (Feinberg 2001) presented it as a continuum was the first time I had heard that and so it is kinda strange, but then if you think about it, it makes total sense. Everything about us biomedically, physically, is on a continuum and so why wouldn't that be also? But it was so appalling to me that I'd never heard of it I mean just on a daily basis, I would never had thought that it was a regular issue that people had to deal with on a day to day basis and that they were being refused treatment, you know I'm still back in the dark ages where I'm still being appalled that lesbians and gays get treated badly, so I can't imagine what it would be like to have to go through life with this issue. (Class discussion, Shannon Case, Graduate Student, Occupational Therapy)

From an anthropological perspective, homophobia and heterosexism perpetuate old stereotypes and create new ones reflective of local political/economic/moral situations. The extant social ideas regarding gender identities play into the creation of stigmas in precise ways that can be studied and addressed within the purview of clinical medical anthropology training. Stigma, as Goffman (1963) described it, can be something one is born with or something one acquires. According to cultural norms and local contexts, stigmatizing conditions may be revealed or not to different individuals with different degrees of social distance and with various ramifications–everything from social shunning to secondary gains associated with the particular condition (Waxler 1981). Issues of discrimination, subordination and relative privilege within a clinical setting are fundamental theoretical and descriptive issues to be addressed as one intellectually questions the enactment of biomedicine within clinical situations.

In the Clinical Medical Anthropology class, films are used to give specific examples of issues such as this. One particularly effective film, *You Don't Know Dick*, explores the lifeworlds of women who have sex changes and subsequently live their lives as men. How these individuals reveal their need to engage in hormonal and surgical treatments, who they talk to, the responses of family, friends and medical professionals, are all poignantly described in the interviews that comprise this documentary film. The issue of engaging in this sort of medical treatment as well as the discrimination and social shunning that these individuals face is shocking to many of the students. Films engage students and give them the chance to apply anthropological concepts.

GENDERIZING UNDERSTANDINGS OF CLINICIANS

Clinical worlds are peopled not just with patients but also with clinicians. While oft-ignored, the lifeworlds of clinicians leak over into their biomedical work. Not simply enforcers of medical regimen and protocols, clinicians bring with them all their own preconceived notions, stereotypes and ideas of gender identity. Cassell (1998) describes surgeons working within large hospitals from a gender perspective. She demonstrates how the way that one "does gender" can play a defining role in the enactment of patient care.

> Cassell's book not only tells about the individual experiences of women surgeons, but of the greater context, that of living as a surgeon in a woman's body. Society has placed values on gender that inhibit the ability to act as a surgeon. Women (surgeons) are seen as too masculine or too feminine, both of which are unacceptable. (Sheri Murphy, Undergraduate Nursing Student, class memo 10/2/01)

Ethnographies such as Cassell's (1998) bring clinical reality within the reach of students who may have little clinical experience themselves. As one student commented in her weekly class memo:

People, including surgeons, "do" gender, and they "are" female–they begin to embody knowledge the day they are born. This theory encompasses a gut feeling that we all have that we are acting naturally (unconsciously) and fluidly from day to day–that we have a unique identity (as a result of our personal interactions), but are, at the same time, a member of a symbolic and physically manifested group. This group is at times at odds with "others," and at times struggles within itself to maintain/push at its borders, to question/support the place of the group within a larger social system. These contradictions exist, partly because the current socio-cultural climate (which superficially supports women's ascension to high-level, powerful positions, while relegating the majority to traditionally submissive roles) allows, even encourages [these contradictions to exist]. (Heather Schaper, Graduate Student, Medical Anthropology, class memo 10/23/01)

Beyond examples of women trying to break gender-role expectations by choosing to work in traditionally male-dominated occupations like surgery, other, basic issues about workday rhythms and timing can be called into question. Even within professions dominated by women such as midwifery, gender role expectations clash with job expectations. In their description of midwives working in the socialized medical system of the United Kingdom, Wrede, Benoit and Sandall discuss how midwives were forced to choose between being with their families or working extraordinarily long hours. New patterns of care contained an inherent assumption about the "genderless" job, which required flexibility and availability and ignored the needs of almost half the midwifery workforce who had young children at home (2001:34). Through the use of such case studies, students are exposed to sufficient local details to begin to ask similar questions in a variety of cross-cultural clinical settings. The act of being able to envisage new "paradigms of professional practice" rests on expanding the imagination to encompass possible solutions to such things as the highly structured and sometimes inhumane learning strategies in medical schools and residency programs (Good 1995).

Bourdieu gives clinical medical anthropologists a way in which to conceptually describe and theorize about ways of learning and enacting specialized knowledge that goes beyond the codified, written representations that appear in medical textbooks. He challenges us to think about the unconscious and unquestioning embodied performances of clinicians in medical institutions (e.g., Cartwright 1998). Students can begin to envision new paradigms of professional practice that do not take for granted 12 or 24 hour shifts or months on end of work without vacations. It becomes apparent that male and female clinicians of all gender persuasions could provide services that would be healthier and perhaps even more efficacious for their clientele if they were not forced into extremely long hours of work and unremitting exhaustion. Whether or not future generations of practitioners replicate existing, rigid notions of the work day and the sexual division of labor in the home, depends, at least in part, on students being exposed to other possible paradigms of living and working in the 21st century. Things such as paternal leave for the birth of a child and flexible clinician work hours seem obvious starting points.

Both clinicians and patients engage in their lives via their gender identities and those that are in non-traditional unions have needs and experiences that have barely been touched by medical anthropologists. Ragoné and Twine (2000) have begun to question some of these experiences with respect to motherhood, but a vast universe of other gender issues and biomedical realms outside obstetrics await study.

> Balance will not be achieved until the issue of gender is taken up as a serious area of concern. The issue must be approached in a way that is palatable to the entire spectrum of negotiated and embodied gender identities.
> (Diana Campanella, Graduate Student, Medical Anthropology, class 10/23/01)

The next section of the class focused on applying clinical medical anthropology concepts to particular diseases.

DIAGNOSIS AND FOREKNOWLEDGE: DILEMMAS INHERENT IN TRYING TO PREDICT THE FUTURE AND VINDICATE THE PAST

There are clinical moments that are very difficult to convey to students who do not have experience working directly with patients. These moments, such as when a practitioner must convey the diagnosis of a very serious, perhaps incurable illness, are quintessentially important to the understanding of the workings of clinical settings. These moments are often lost when it comes to writing up research findings in journal articles and monographs. Some of the best descriptions come from fictional or semi-fictional writing such as in the following account. I include this extended quote from an assigned class reading as an elegant sample of writing that takes students out of their everyday worlds and into a mind-space where they can react emotionally. Many of them are clinicians in training and they are given few chances to explore the affective side of working in and around clinics in their programs of study.

> The first few seconds were like an ecstasy, a rapture, so pure I almost wasn't there. I'm writing this down because it's a moment our friends

don't speak of, our writers don't write about. Characters in books, our husbands, neighbours, aunts, float in from the wings already knowing, already changed. It's a moment of such solitude, such nakedness, so utterly unlike any other, that we tend to look away from it politely as from an obscenity. If it is obscene it's because it leaves us shamelessly stripped of our learnt humanity, as animal, as instinctual as any monkey. Yet it's a moment that comes in the end to almost everyone.

Then I imploded. Some people probably explode at this point, bursting into tears, awash with anger and regret and fear and impotence. I can imagine, too, desperately want to drag time backwards just by a second or two and rerun the scene with different dialogue, no, before it's too late: "it looks like that flu that's going around . . . the wooziness, the lack of appetite . . . Take a few days off, I'll write you out a prescription . . ." Please say it again like that. Please. That did flash through my mind. But the seconds ticked on, carrying me with them. And I imploded. (Dessaix 1996:6-7)

"Listening in" to this situation of a patient being told he has HIV/AIDS is a powerful emotional and intellectual event. Like the character in Dessaix's (1996) book *Night Letters*, and indeed like the author himself, we witness conditions like AIDS and cancer and other illnesses that imply fundamental shifts in how individuals think about the remaining days and hours of their lives. Writing on the boundary of fiction and non-fiction, the writer Robert Dessaix uses his illness and gender experiences to explore what such diagnoses mean. His writing involves students emotionally and allows them to challenge sterile clinical descriptions of topics such as "doctor-patient communication" and "stigmatization."

In this section of the class we use the concepts and theoretical constructs from the first part of the semester (illness narratives, conversation analysis, stigma, risk, etc.) to explore particular configurations of issues that surround diagnoses such as AIDS, cancer, late onset neurogenetic diseases like amyotrophic lateral sclerosis (Lou Gerhig's disease), and environmentally-induced illnesses (Balshem 1993). The students explore each disease from different levels–the individual, the social and the larger socio-economic context (Scheper-Hughes and Lock 1987, Kaufert 2000), using the analytical frameworks developed by the authors already discussed in class. From genetic testing (Rapp 1999), through diagnosis, treatment and beyond, the class explores different clinical scenarios. The creative intellectual work comes in taking the theories and applying them to different clinical settings and to different disease states; students work up individual written term papers in this manner.

CONCLUSIONS

In this essay I have not tried to cover the entire literature of clinical medical anthropology that pertains to gender issues, but have instead focused on a progression of topics that seems to me to take students through the intellectual and emotional steps necessary to begin to question and research gender relations in the clinical setting. Often, it is a most difficult task to see what is right before one's eyes, to challenge beloved notions of things like "the family doctor" and the power and hope of biomedicine. While in some cases these constructs need no challenging, there are also many times when they do. To provide students with "different hats" to put on with respect to the socially constructed nature of gender may well be a way to continue the process of making biomedicine an institution that can best serve both the patients who seek to be healed and the clinicians who spend their lives working to heal them.

REFERENCES

Balshem, M. (1993). *Cancer in the Community: Class and Medical Authority*, Smithsonian Institution Press, Washington and London.

Becker, G. (1997). *Disrupted Lives: How People Create Meaning in a Chaotic World*, University of California Press, Berkeley.

Bishop, E. (1984). *Elizabeth Bishop, The Complete Poems, 1927-1979*, Farrar, Straus, Giroux, New York.

Bourdieu, P. (1990). *The Logic of Practice*, Stanford University Press, Stanford, CA.

Cartwright, E. (1998). *"The Logic of Heartbeats: Electronic Fetal Monitoring and Biomedically Constructed Birth"* (pp. 240-254), in ed. R. Davis-Floyd and J. Dumit *Cyborg Babies: From Techno-Sex to Techno-Tots*, Routledge, New York

Cartwright, E. and J. Thomas (2001). *"Constructing Risk: Maternity Care, Law, and Malpractice"* (pp. 203-217) in ed. Devries, R., Benoit, C., Van Teijlingen, E. and S. Wrede, *Birth By Design: Pregnancy, Maternity Care, and Midwifery in North America and Europe*, Routledge, New York.

Cassell, J. (1998). *The Woman in the Surgeon's Body*, Harvard University Press, Cambridge, MA and London, England.

Davis-Floyd, R. (1992). *Birth as an American Rite of Passage*, University of California Press, Berkeley.

Dessaix, R. (1996). *Night Letters*, Saint Martin's Press, New York.

Devries, R., Benoit, C., Van Teijlingen, E. and S. Wrede (2001). *Birth By Design: Pregnancy, Maternity Care, and Midwifery in North America and Europe*, Routledge, New York.

Dillard, A. (1999). *For the Time Being*, Knopf, New York.

Douglas, M. (1992). *Risk and Blame: Essays in Cultural Theory*, Routledge, New York.

Feinberg, L. (2001). *"Trans Health Crisis: For Us It's Life or Death"* American Journal of Public Health 91(6):897-900.

Fisher, S. and A. Todd, eds. (1983). *The Social Organization of Doctor-Patient Communication*, Center for Applied Linguistics, Washington, DC.

Foucault, M. (1973). *The Birth of the Clinic: An Archaeology of Medical Perception*, Vintage Books, New York.

Goffman, E. (1963). *Stigma: Notes on the Management of Spoiled Identity*, Simon and Schuster, New York.

Good, M. (1995). *American Medicine: The Quest for Competence*, University of California Press, Berkeley.

Habermas, J. (1984). *The Theory of Communicative Action, Reason, and the Rationalization of Society* volume 1, Heinemann Press, London.

Hopkins, K. (2001). "*Are Brazilian Women Really Choosing to Deliver by Cesarean?*" Social Science and Medicine 51:725-740.

Kaufert, P. (2000). "*Health Policy and the New Genetics*" Social Science and Medicine 51:821-829.

Le Guin, U. K. (1981). "*It Was a Dark and Stormy Night: Or, Why Are We Huddling About the Campfire?*" in ed. W. Mitchell, *On Narrative*, University of Chicago Press, Chicago.

Meyer, I. H. (2001). "*Why Lesbian, Gay, Bisexual, and Transgender Health?*" American Journal of Public Health 91(6):856-858.

Miller, A. M. (2001). "*Uneasy Promises: Sexuality, Health, and Human Rights*" American Journal of Public Health 91(6):861-864.

Mishler, E. G. (1984). *The Discourse of Medicine. The Dialectics of Medical Interviews*, Ablex Press, Norwood, NJ.

Moerman, M. (1988). *Talking Culture: Ethnography and Conversation Analysis*, University of Pennsylvania Press, Philadelphia.

Polanyi, L. (1981). "*Telling the Same Story Twice*" Text 1(4):315-336.

Price, L. (1987). "*Ecuadorian Illness Stories; Cultural Knowledge in Natural Discourse*" (pp. 313-342) in eds. D. Holland and N. Quinn, *Cultural Models in Language and Thought*, Cambridge University Press, New York.

Ragoné, H. and F. Twine (2000). *Ideologies and Technologies of Motherhood: Race, Class, Sexuality Nationalism*, Routledge, New York.

Rapp, R. (1999). *Testing Women, Testing the Fetus–The Social Impact of Amniocentesis in America*. Routledge, New York.

Sacks, H., Schegloff, E. and G. Jefferson (1974). "*A Simplest Systematics for the Organization of Turn Taking for Conversation*" Language 59(4):696-735.

Scheper-Hughes, N. and M. Lock (1987). "*The Mindful Body: A Prolegomenon to Future Work in Medical Anthropology*" Medical Anthropology Quarterly 1(1):6-41.

Skolbekken, J. (1995). "*The Risk Epidemic in Medical Journals*" Social Science and Medicine 40(3):291-305.

Waxler, N. (1981). "*Learning to Be a Leper: A Case Study in the Social Construction of Illness*" in ed. E. Mishler, *Social Contexts of Health, Illness and Patient Care*, Cambridge University Press, Cambridge.

Wrede, S., Benoit, C. and J. Sandall (2001). "*The State and Birth/The State of Birth: Maternal Health Policy in Three Countries*" (pp. 28-50) in eds. Devries, R., Benoit, C., Van Teijlingen, E. and S. Wrede, *Birth By Design: Pregnancy, Maternity Care, and Midwifery in North America and Europe*, Routledge, New York.

Gender in Medical Curricula: Course Organizer Views of a Gender-Issues Perspective in Medicine in Sweden

Anna Westerståhl, MD, PhD
Maria Andersson, MD, PhD
Margareta Söderström, MD, PhD

SUMMARY. While there is growing awareness of the importance of gender issues in medicine, with new knowledge and new perspectives in-

Anna Westerståhl is General Practitioner in Göteborg, Lecturer and Doctoral Student at the Department of Primary Health Care at Göteborg University. Her teaching of medical students is focused on consultation skills and her research field on issues of gender, sexual orientation and power in medical education and in the consultation. She will present her thesis in 2003. Maria Andersson has recently finished her internship at Malmö University Hospital. Her scientific field is capillary physiology, and she received her PhD from Göteborg University in 2000. There she was also engaged in a gender project in medical education. Margareta Söderström is General Practitioner in Malmö and Senior Lecturer, Department of General Practice, Copenhagen University. Her research field focuses on restorative environments and the health of pre-schoolers, as well as gender perspective issues on medical education and research ethic reviewing.

Address correspondence to: Anna Westerståhl, Sahlgrenska Akademin, Göteborg University, Department of Family Medicine, Box 454, SE-40530 Göteborg, Sweden (E-mail: anna.westerstahl@allmed.gu.se).

The authors acknowledge the support of the Medical Faculty and the Department of Family Medicine at Göteborg University, Sweden. They also acknowledge the valuable comments by Ingrid Toshach Gustafsson, Lecturer at Department of Education at Göteborg University, and Ullaliina Lehtinen, Senior Lecturer at University College of Borås and at Karolinska Institutet, Stockholm.

[Haworth co-indexing entry note]: "Gender in Medical Curricula: Course Organizer Views of a Gender-Issues Perspective in Medicine in Sweden." Westerståhl, Anna, Maria Andersson, and Margareta Söderström. Co-published simultaneously in *Women & Health* (The Haworth Medical Press, an imprint of The Haworth Press, Inc.) Vol. 37, No. 4, 2003, pp. 35-47; and: *Teaching Gender, Teaching Women's Health: Case Studies in Medical and Health Science Education* (ed: Lenore Manderson) The Haworth Medical Press, an imprint of The Haworth Press, Inc., 2003, pp. 35-47. Single or multiple copies of this article are available for a fee from The Haworth Document Delivery Service [1-800-HAWORTH, 9:00 a.m. - 5:00 p.m. (EST). E-mail address: docdelivery@haworthpress.com].

tensely debated, reports on the implementation of gender issues into medical curricula are scarce. In 1996, the Medical Faculty of Göteborg University, Sweden, determined that a gender-issues perspective be included in medical education. In 1999, course organizers from preclinical and clinical departments of the faculty were interviewed to determine whether they felt that a gender-issues perspective had contributed to their scientific field and, if so, how they implemented it in their teaching. The interviews revealed varied opinions on the relevance of this perspective in medicine. These variations followed gender division rather than that of preclinicians/clinicians. Thus, female gender was overwhelming for inspiring and introducing a gender-issues perspective both scientifically and practically. Positivism is firmly established in medicine and this must be taken into consideration when introducing a more culturally- and socially-based understanding of sex/gender issues. Female gender is important in this process, but successful implementation requires thorough faculty support and participation of male colleagues and students. *[Article copies available for a fee from The Haworth Document Delivery Service: 1-800-HAWORTH. E-mail address: <docdelivery@haworthpress.com> Website: <http://www.HaworthPress.com> © 2003 by The Haworth Press, Inc. All rights reserved.]*

KEYWORDS. Gender, women's health, implementation, medical education, curriculum

INTRODUCTION

The expanding literature on women's health and/or gender issues is impressive. Biological sex differences have been lifted out of formerly sex-blind contexts, and traditional medical health concepts have been expanded with social theories (Hurtley & Benditt, 1995; Rönnberg & Hammarström, 2000). Thus, the traditional view of the 70 kg white male as the normative research subject or patient is no longer accepted. At the same time, society's evolving expectations of medical practitioners have resulted in new approaches to medical research and education throughout the world. Medical faculties are now expected to train future physicians in a manner that sensitises them to issues of gender, ethnicity and other perspectives relevant to increasingly complex societies (Kuntz, 1997). The medical literature on these issues sometimes reflects controversies of the concepts of sex and gender. "Gender" and "women's health" are used alternatively, and sex differences, e.g., in brain anatomy, are sometimes described as gender differences. Women's health is not synonymous with gender (health), however, even if women as a marginalized group have had an interest in drawing attention to their neglected needs. Gender comprises both men and women, and there is today an increasing body of research on masculinity, often with a feminist starting point (Connell, 1995). Also, from a political and conceptual point of view, the emphasis on the difference between sex and gender, between body and social context, has been pivotal in helping to avoid biologism. In the medical context, the emphasis on sex/gender difference is still important, but requires a sharply defined partition between the body and the social context, a presumption that is increasingly challenged by other sciences (Shildrick & Price, 1998). The literature on incorporating a gender perspective into medical education is scarce, but bears witness to the difficulties in ongoing curriculum changes (Searle, 1998; Robinson & Stewart, 1996). Notwithstanding both theoretical and practical difficulties, the Medical Faculty of the University of Göteborg decided in 1996 that a gender-issues perspective be included in medical education whenever appropriate. No instructions of how this might occur followed and there was no plan for evaluation. Therefore, in 1999 and on our own initiative, we decided to interview course organizers in the Medical Faculty to find out whether they considered that a gender perspective had added anything to their scientific field, and if so, how they implemented it in their teaching.

METHOD

An invitation to participate in a telephone interview was sent to all course organizers of major subject fields at the medical faculty (N = 26). If a course organizer declined, she/he was asked to suggest another informant from that department. The telephone interviews were semi-structured, allowing for the informant to expand her/his ideas and for the interviewer to ask for clarification (Table 1). If requested, a definition of "a gender-issues perspective" was provided, which included aspects of both sex and gender (in Swedish, there is a single, common word, *kön*, that covers both concepts). If further clarification was requested, examples of new insights into coronary heart disease were given (Schenk-Gustafsson, 1996). The three authors participated equally in the interviews, which lasted between 15 minutes and one hour. Keywords were noted during the interviews, notes from which were expanded and sent back to the informants, who were invited to correct the text or add to it. Most interviews were returned unchanged or with minor factual errors corrected, but one informant had cut out half his interview. When all the interviews were complete, the participant course organizers were invited to a seminar to discuss the preliminary results.

The text was analysed using a descriptive/analytical approach (Malterud, 1996). Descriptive codes were created through joint close-text reading, and were then sorted into more theoretical categories. Some of these categories formed the basis of core concepts, which were also influenced by the interview context and the seminar. Less common and unusual responses and comments were sorted into groups of answers or merely described.

RESULTS

Interviews were conducted with 67% of the male and 75% of the female course organizers, comprising 7 preclinicians and 19 clinicians (Table 2). While the focus of the study lay on issues of knowledge and implementation, the results drew attention also to the impact of learning, and this forms the second of the two core concepts presented below.

Contribution to Knowledge

Many of the clinical course organizers said that there was new knowledge in their scientific field and gave examples from their own daily work with patients (Table 3). These examples included living conditions as well as behav-

TABLE 1. Main Questions Asked in Interviews

1. Has the current discussion (scientific or popular) of a gender-issues perspective in medicine supplied new knowledge to your medical speciality?

2. If so, how do you implement it in your teaching?

3. What about the students? Do they ask about gender issues in medicine? Are there any differences between male and female students?

4. How did you learn about gender issues?

5. Are you interested in learning more about how to teach with a gender-issues perspective?

TABLE 2. Informants According to Gender and Academic Affiliation

	Preclinicians n (%)*	Clinicians n (%)*	Total n (%)*
Male	6 (23)	14 (54)	20 (77)
Female	1 (4)	5 (19)	6 (23)
Total	7 (27)	19 (73)	26 (100)

*Proportion of total number (N = 26) of informants

TABLE 3. Opinions of Gender in Medicine Forming the Core Concept of *Diversity and Boundaries*. Citations from Clinicians in Italics, from Preclinicians in Plain Text

Citations about knowledge	Description of a gender-issues perspective as ...	Scientific standpoint
My field is theoretical–we ask questions independently of gender and as natural scientists we aim at objectivity	Practical and subjective (biased)	
Gender has no relevance in my field so the content is not loaded with that perspective	Irrelevant and/or disadvantageous	
Our field has had enough trouble with becoming accepted...		
It is comfortable to be able to have a purely scientific attitude toward one's field	Uncomfortable and unscientific	Different from (natural) science and/or problematic
There is a difference between male and female brains, and I know that is a controversial issue	Biologically founded but controversial when it comes to conclusions	
From our studies on rats we try to understand gender differences in addiction development	Founded on biological differences	
Behavioural differences between boys and girls due to neonatal trouble are purely biological		
To understand gender differences in living conditions is of vital importance when working with serious illness	Crucial in some (serious) aspects of clinical work	
Through my close work with female patients I have learnt so much about what it is to be a woman	Expanding clinical knowledge (about women)	
For some diagnoses, gender differences in prevalence are due to different ways of living		Integrated in the application of science and obvious

TABLE 3 (continued)

Citations about knowledge	Description of a gender-issues perspective as . . .	Scientific standpoint
There is a gender difference in the way men and women talk about their lives	Important and obvious knowledge for everyday clinical work	Integrated in the application of science and obvious
Gender differences are very much about differences in working and home conditions		
It is unbelievable the things we used to claim about sex differences concerning ECG diagnosis		

ioral problems, which they considered to be biologically founded. The few informants who did not see any relevance of gender said that their patients were individuals, not gendered, or that the perspective was relevant but disadvantageous to their speciality. Most of the preclinical course organizers said that there was no new knowledge, as their subject was gender-neutral. Some mentioned sex differences at a molecular level. They said they welcomed a gender perspective, and explained its absence to lack of female colleagues. They also raised equality issues in the faculty, including problems of sexual harassment in their own and other departments. A number of interviews also drew attention to the need for demarcation lines between objectivity and science on the one hand and subjectivity and non-science on the other. This dichotomy, while not necessarily associated with gender or academic affiliation of informants, sheds light on the *diversity and boundaries within medical education*, and formed the first of the two core concepts in the present study (again, see Table 3).

Implementation in Teaching

There was scarce information about teaching with a gender perspective, and the answers could best be sorted into four groups. The first group consisted of informants who had never used a gender perspective because of perceived lack of relevance or because they had not thought about it. The second group wanted to use a gender perspective but did not do so because of (self-perceived) lack of skills, knowledge or collegial support. The third group taught biological differences between the sexes, as they had always done, but some had become more aware of the importance of this or now felt that a biological perspective was too restrictive. The fourth group, mainly in epidemiology, taught gender differences in living conditions and health behaviour and considered this unproblematic. A few clinicians in this group also brought up issues of gender differences in patients' use of language, compliance and the like interactions with the students.

According to most informants, teaching biological sex differences was easily accepted by the students. Teaching gender issues was more problematic because it sometimes evoked feelings of resentment or anger in students. Male students especially sometimes thought that the teaching was too focused on women. Female students were reported to be more interested in learning about gender than male students, and also were able to involve themselves more deeply in discussions and give much more balanced contributions. A few stated that the students never asked for a gender-issues perspective. The explanations given were that the students were ignorant, had no interest in discussing the matter, or that the perspective was not relevant.

Talking to academic staff about students generated many comments concerning different gender characteristics of students (Table 4). Most of the perceived characteristics of female students were considered beneficial, while the characteristics of male students were negatively loaded. Informants explained these differences as "probably genetic," but they also acknowledged factors in upbringing. A few of the course organizers felt that there were few differences between male and female students, and a greater variation between different classes of students or different ethnic groups.

Learning About Gender Issues

Many male course organizers had gained awareness of gender issues from discussions at home, and the underlying notion was that they learned about gender issues by living close to women (Table 5). Only one of the female teachers mentioned her husband, and a few declared that you "learn by living" (as women). Some informants said that they had learned from long experience with patients, especially with women. Female colleagues were of utmost importance in raising gender issues, and in male-only departments, discussion related to gender did not take place unless necessary. Other sources of information were female writers and journalists, and two informants (a man and a woman) had attended academic courses on gender-related issues. The dominant sources of knowledge about gender issues therefore were the private sphere or daily work, through a personal experience as or with women. Thus, *female gender as the source of knowledge* forms the second of the core concepts in the present study. Some of the informants said that they had not learnt anything about gender issues at all, or that they did not know or understand anything about the subject.

TABLE 4. Perceived Differences Between Female and Male Medical Students as Reported by Course Organizers

Female students	Male students
Sensitive	Silent
Listening	Capable
Comprehensive	Forward Looking
Cautious	Goal Oriented
Scrupulous	Careless
Anxious	Blokish
Careful	
Balanced	
Profound	
Mature	
Soft	
Ambitious	
Eager to Learn	
Reliable	
Robust	
Skilled	
Capable	

Improving Teaching

A quarter of the course organizers (and five out of six of the women) wanted to learn more about gender issues, half of them said yes with reservations, and a quarter said no. Lack of time was the most common obstacle to attending new courses. A few male informants said that such education should be of high standard, with lectures held by well-known lecturers, so that other prioritized assignments could be put aside. Female informants with previous experience of teaching wanted to improve their teaching methods, since the subject of gender often aroused controversy among the students.

Follow-Up Seminar

Six course organizers attended the seminar at which the preliminary results were presented. Much of the discussion was about defining the issue, and one

TABLE 5. Experiences of Learning Forming the Core Concept of *Female Gender as the Source of Knowledge*. Citations by Male Informants in Italics, by Female Informants in Plain Text

Citations about own learning	Learning circumstances	Prerequisite/who was she?
I have been a woman all my life!	Being a woman	Female gender
I have learnt a lot through my wife	Having a wife	Women in family
I am married!		
I grew up with a feminist; that is my mother	Having a mother	
I have a daughter and I have been thinking a lot about her future	Having daughters	
I have two sisters who work as doctors	Having sisters	
I have read books by EW and EK, and I read journals	Reading fiction, biographies, or self studies of scientific reports	Well known female feminist writers, journalists, researchers
I recently read NB and although she is young I appreciate her standpoint		
I have read UH's study on gender and education		
I usually listen to Freja (a daily radio programme) when I drive home	Using media reports	
I contacted AW and CW just after the publication of their article in Daily News		
There are two female colleagues at our department and they are very much aware of gender issues	Taking part in everyday work	Female feminist colleagues in education, at department
You know that I work close to CB and AS, so the gender perspective is always there		
The things that happened when I was a member of the Medical Research Board made me, although late, reflect	Having special assignments	

TABLE 5 (continued)

Citations about own learning	Learning circumstances	Prerequisite/who was she?
I attended a residency course on psychosocial issues with BW	Attending mandatory courses	Female feminist colleagues in education, at department
I have learnt especially from AW who makes her message clearly understandable	Attending faculty meetings	

informant asked for a "gold standard" for gender issues in medicine. It was also suggested that some of the responses were "politically correct" in order to follow the guidelines of the faculty and because of the (female) gender of the interviewers. It was implicit in this suggestion that an honest answer would have been much more hostile to the relevance of gender issues.

DISCUSSION

Method

Telephone interviews, compared with personal in depth interviews, have the advantage of being efficient and easy to conduct, offering a possibility to reach a larger number of informants. The disadvantages are less close contact with the informant and difficulty in catching all that is said. There is also a risk of introducing one's own values and understanding into the transcript. In the present study, we tried to diminish these disadvantages by inviting the informants to comment on the interview transcripts and to take part in a follow-up seminar. Having done this, the analysis proceeded with the concentrated text mainly relying on keywords (e.g., the adjectives in Table 4) combined with short verbatim citations. Budget restrictions limited our ability to interview all course organizers, but all major subject fields were covered.

Diversity and Boundaries

The varied curriculum of medical education is reflected in the present study. The inclusion of a gender perspective makes the curriculum even more difficult to define. Lent and Bishop suggest eight dimensions of gender issues that could be introduced into medical curricula (Lent & Bishop, 1998). Some of these dimensions, e.g., different life experiences, different presentation of problems and risk factors, were mentioned by our informants. Other dimensions, e.g., violence in intimate relationships, were not mentioned. Zelek et al. (1997) presented guidelines for assessing the gender sensitivity of curricula comprising content, language and process, but these detailed instructions would require an advanced awareness of gender issues in faculty. Our study showed that gender sensitivity was scattered, relying on individual reflections and interests.

The subject of gender issues provoked feelings of exclusion and unease as well as applause and recognition. The reason for exclusion was the strongly held opinion that science is objective and pure, compared with gender issues, and this was also reflected in the wish for a "gold standard." The purity of science was described as comfortable, a place in which to rest and be safe. Such preserving of boundaries has been described as barriers to implementing broad curricula (Searle, 1998). The objectivity criterion has also been criticized by many authors (Fausto-Sterling, 1992). The unease experienced by many respondents is also important, as is the opinion that a gender perspective might be disadvantageous to a discipline. This implies that suggestions and guidelines from the faculty are required. Searle (1998) also describes the importance of support from students, provided that they are invited to take an active part in a change of curriculum.

For some informants, the relevance of a gender-issues perspective was evident. Others understood it as an adding of biological news on sex differences, as if they had merely been forgotten. We think that it is essential to remember that the neglect of women's health issues has been and is due to power structures and the different valuation of men and women in society. The abundance of literature on coronary heart disease in women has not been followed by anything similar from other clinical disciplines, and only a few of the informants in the present study mentioned any such need for new knowledge. We regard it a very reasonable hypothesis, that sex and gender differences work in all disciplines, and that the real task is to show where they are of no relevance.

Gender Stereotypes

The perceived difference between female and male students is without doubt an empirically-based experience of many informants. But it also comes close to what is generally regarded as typical female and male characteristics, and this in turn may have a heavy impact on the expectations of as well as feedback to the students. Research has shown the dominant influence on behaviour of the teachers' gender-biased attitudes, and to change attitudes is difficult (Månsson, 2000). It is worth noting that in our study, informants were more likely to attribute comments to female students than the male students. These attributions were mainly positive, and it is possible that the growing number of women in medical studies has contributed to structural change. But when discussions about gender issues occur, and female students are addressed, they are sometimes considered to dominate the scene by both men and women. Our experience as teachers is also that female students may feel singled out as "losers"–i.e., that subordination is inevitable–and male students feel a sense of guilt when gender issues are discussed (Westerståhl & Björkelund, 1998).

Gender Is Also About and for Men

An impressive result of the finding was the almost mandatory presence of female gender–either by being a woman or serving as a role model and providing inspiration for the informants' learning about gender. There is nothing surprising that women, as a marginalized group, speak for themselves, and the difficulties and shortcomings of academic women have been convincingly analysed (Wennerås & Wold, 1997). But gender issues are about women *and* men, and if men do not take an active part in discussing them, there is a risk of maintaining the status quo, or regarding the gender issues as of secondary importance.

It is also thought-provoking to note that the private sphere and daily work-relations were so important as sources of learning about gender issues in science (a question asked by interviewers). While this might be where gender awareness starts, there is an urgent need for scientifically-based knowledge about how gender works in medicine.

CONCLUSION

Who knows about and who teaches gender issues in medicine? According to our study, there was an overwhelming dominance of hard working women in the academy and elsewhere to introduce and inspire a gender perspective. The time has come for a change, however, and male colleagues need to take part in this boundary-transgressing activity to elucidate the concept of gender.

What is and what will be taught about gender issues? Our study underlines the diversity of the medical curriculum, which requires diversity in content as well as in form of teaching. The strict positivistic standpoint is a reality in medicine and demands attention when introducing a more culturally- and socially-based understanding of sex/gender issues. The results also emphasize that individual enthusiasm is not enough. Faculty policies must be prepared, followed up, and, as others have shown, carried forward by students.

REFERENCES

Connell, R. (1995). *Masculinities: knowledge, power, and social change.* Berkeley: University of California Press.

Fausto-Sterling, A. (1992). *Myths of gender. Biological theories about women and men.* New York: Basic Books: Harper Collins.

Hurtley, S., Benditt, J. (1995). Women's health research. Special issue. *Science*, 269, 766-800.

Kuntz, C. (1997). Medical curricula for the next millennium: responding to diversity. *Canadian Medical Association Journal*, 156, 1295-1296.

Lent B., Bishop J. (1998). Sense and sensitivity: Developing a gender-issues perspective in medical education. *Journal of Women's Health*, 7, 339-342.

Malterud, K. (1996). *Kvalitativa metoder i medicinsk forskning. En innföring (Qualitative methods in medical research. An introduction)*. Aurskog, Norge: Tano Aschehoug (pp. 87-104).

Månsson, A. (2000). *Gendered encounters–Pattern of interaction in nursery schools between preschool staff and small children in a gendered perspective*. Thesis. Reprocentralen, Lärarutbildningen. Lund University.

Robinson, G., Stewart D. (1996). A curriculum on physician-patient sexual misconduct and teacher-learner mistreatment. Part 1: Content and Part 2: Teaching method. *CMAJ*, 154, 643-649 and 1021-1025.

Rönnberg A., Hammarström A. (2000). Barriers within the health care system to dealing with sexualized violence: a literature review. *Scand J Public Health*, 28, 222-229.

Schenk-Gustafsson, K. (1996). Risk factors for cardiovascular disease in women. Assessments and management. *Eur Heart J*, 17(Suppl D), 2-8.

Shildrick M., Price J. (1998). In M. Shildrick & J. Price (eds). *Vital Signs–Feminist Reconfiguration of the Bio/logical Body* (pp 1-17). Edinburgh. Edinburgh University Press.

Searle J. (1998). Introduction of a new curriculum in women's health in medical education: a framework for change. *Women's Health Issues*, 8, 382-388.

Wennerås C., Wold A. (1997). Nepotism and sexism in peer review. *Nature*, 387, 341-343.

Westerståhl A., Björkelund C. (1998). Medical students became aware of a gender perspective. *Läkartidningen*, 16, 1817-1819.

Zelek, B., Phillips, S., Lefebvre, Y. (1997). Gender sensitivity in medical curricula. *Can Med Assoc J*, 156, 1297-1300.

Women Teaching Women's Health: Issues in the Establishment of a Clinical Teaching Associate Program for the Well Woman Check

Kathryn Robertson, MBBS, MEd   Vivienne O'Connor, MBChB
Kelsey Hegarty, MBBS, PhD   Jane Gunn, MBBS, PhD

Kathryn Robertson is General Practitioner, Director of the Clinical Teaching Associate Program and Coordinator of the Simulated Patient Program, Department of General Practice, University of Melbourne, Melbourne, Australia. She brings to these roles extensive experience in undergraduate and postgraduate medical education, particularly in the fields of communication skills, doctor-patient relationships and the Patient-Centred Approach. She completed her Masters of Education with a thesis on the use of Simulated Patients in the teaching and assessment of communication skills for medical students. Kelsey Hegarty is an academic general practitioner who has general interests in women's health, in particular women's emotional wellbeing. Her research experience includes a doctoral thesis on measurement and prevalence of partner abuse in general practice and projects on depression and counselling. She is interested in further exploring the barriers to disclosure of sensitive issues in general practice. She has had extensive teaching experience at undergraduate and postgraduate levels in the areas of women's health, mental health and advanced communication skills. Vivienne O'Connor is Senior Lecturer in Obstetrics and Gynaecology, University of Queensland. She initiated the Clinical Teaching Associate Program for the University of Queensland in 1996, initially funded by a grant from the Queensland Cancer Fund and subsequently taken over by the University. She teaches in the MBBS Program and the Graduate Health Studies Program. Vivienne convenes the annual women's health conference for general practitioners which will be in its tenth year in 2003. She is co-editing a textbook on Women's Health for publication in 2003. Jane Gunn is Research Director, Department of General Practice, University of Melbourne. She is involved in women's health research in primary care, with a particular interest in the health of mothers. Her research combines qualitative and quantitative methods. She is actively involved in teaching medical students and has expertise in the use of simulated patients in teaching and research.

Address correspondence to: Dr. Kathryn Robertson, Department of General Practice, University of Melbourne, 200 Berkeley Street, Carlton, VIC 3053, Australia (E-mail: k.robertson@unimelb.edu.au).

[Haworth co-indexing entry note]: "Women Teaching Women's Health: Issues in the Establishment of a Clinical Teaching Associate Program for the Well Woman Check." Robertson, Kathryn et al. Co-published simultaneously in *Women & Health* (The Haworth Medical Press, an imprint of The Haworth Press, Inc.) Vol. 37, No. 4, 2003, pp. 49-65; and: *Teaching Gender, Teaching Women's Health: Case Studies in Medical and Health Science Education* (ed: Lenore Manderson) The Haworth Medical Press, an imprint of The Haworth Press, Inc., 2003, pp. 49-65. Single or multiple copies of this article are available for a fee from The Haworth Document Delivery Service [1-800-HAWORTH, 9:00 a.m. - 5:00 p.m. (EST). E-mail address: docdelivery@haworthpress.com].

10.1300/J013v37n04_05

SUMMARY. The impact of screening programs for cervical cancer would be increased with the greater participation of currently under-screened women. Training for medical students and doctors in the fine technical and communication skills required in breast and gynaecological examinations would improve participation by increasing the confidence and skill of doctors in raising the issue of screening, thereby making the examination a more positive experience for women. Gynaecology Teaching Associate (GTA) programs, using specially trained standardized patients, have been used in over 90% of American and Canadian medical schools for more than ten years to provide such training. Australia has been slow to adopt this teaching method. A Clinical Teaching Associates in Gynaecology program (CTA) was first established in 1996 by the Department of Obstetrics and Gynaecology at the University of Queensland, building on the Pap test program from Adelaide. Other medical schools subsequently introduced such programs and in 2000, the Department of General Practice, University of Melbourne, established a CTA program based on the Queensland program, with a grant from PapScreen Victoria. This paper describes the methods of recruitment and training of CTAs, use of CTAs in the medical course, preliminary evaluation, and ethical and other issues in the Melbourne and Queensland University programs. *[Article copies available for a fee from The Haworth Document Delivery Service: 1-800-HAWORTH. E-mail address: <docdelivery@haworthpress.com> Website: <http://www.HaworthPress.com> © 2003 by The Haworth Press, Inc. All rights reserved.]*

KEYWORDS. Gynaecology, Pap test, sensitive gynaecological examination, communication skills, education, medical, gynaecological teaching associates

INTRODUCTION

All medical examinations are potentially distressing. For women, examinations involving breast and genitalia are particularly intrusive (Moore, 2000). Women require a medical practitioner to be not only technically competent but also sensitive to issues that concern them about such examinations. Medical students do not feel adequately trained in these areas (Lurie, 1998). The clinical teaching associate program was developed to provide a relaxed, professional learning environment to enable students to develop these skills. Clinical teaching associates (CTAs) are women specifically trained to provide guidance and feedback to medical students regarding both the practical and interpersonal skills required in breast and gynaecological examinations, whilst themselves being examined. This provides the foundation to improve all aspects of good practice for the benefit of women undergoing intimate examinations (Beckmann, 1988).

In this paper, we focus on the development of the Well Woman Check tutorials for the University of Melbourne fifth year medical students undertaking obstetrics and gynaecology training, and the student response to the program. For example, students stated that [it] helped with how to reassure and address women and ensure respect and empowerment are maintained.

The University of Melbourne program was based on that developed at the University of Queensland for the MBBS course. The majority of Australian medical schools have at some stage utilized programs similar to that of Queensland University but their development and evaluation have not been published.

BACKGROUND

Why Do We Need to Teach Sensitive Pap Testing?

Regular screening of women at risk is believed to be the key to early detection of cervical cancer (NHMRC, 1997). Many barriers prevent women from presenting for regular Pap tests, however, including lack of knowledge; economic, logistic and social barriers, and embarrassment and fear (Straton, 1994). Pap tests can be physically and emotionally uncomfortable, and women can feel very vulnerable, because of the nature of the position for the test (Alexander, 1981; Lang, 1990; Moore, 2000). One-quarter of the women in one NSW study (Shelley, 1991) said that Pap tests were too uncomfortable and embarrassing to have regularly.

The characteristics of the doctor play an important role in whether women participate in screening. Only 30-40% of women stated that they preferred a female provider (Straton, 1994). Other issues that significantly influence the decision to have regular Pap tests include perceived ease of access, approachability and past screening experiences, particularly with regard to dignity and comfort (Hill, 1985; Fernbach, 1999). Women overdue for screening are likely to rely on their doctor to suggest the test (Cockburn, 1992). Specific training to increase the confidence and skills of doctors will improve the communication and technical aspects of undertaking a sensitive examination and should positively impact on the uptake of screening (Evans et al., 1992; Straton, 1994; Goertzen, 1995).

Currently, medical trainees believe that they are poorly prepared for and uncomfortable while performing sex-sensitive examinations (Lurie, 1998). Lewis showed that many general practitioners have had inadequate training in Pap test taking and that some general practitioners take very few Pap tests (Lewis, 1994). It is reasonable to conclude that medical students and some doctors could be better prepared to take Pap tests sensitively (Taylor, 1997; Ward, 1997; Kann, 1998).

Characteristics of Sensitive Pap Testing

In a Melbourne survey (N = 472), 94.9% of women expressed the need to be informed about what the doctor is doing during the examination (Grindley, 1998; Moore, 2000). The women surveyed were sensitive to comments made by the doctor, and their response varied if the doctor was male or female (Moore, 2000). In another study (N = 977), women stated that they would prefer the use of warm instruments and a gentle examination, and explanation of the procedure while it is being performed (Petravage, 1979). Based on a small qualitative study of recent NSW graduates (N = 23), Ward et al. (1997) outlined several specific interactional behaviours that might reduce the anxieties and discomforts associated with Pap tests. These included providing an explanation about the procedure, establishing permission and a mechanism to stop, explaining how to follow up the result, and offering written information when appropriate.

Training

The Gynaecology Teaching Associate (GTA) instructional method uses standardised patients to teach gynaecological clinical skills, and has been used overseas in over 90% of American and Canadian medical schools (Beckmann, 1988). Standardized, or simulated, patients (SPs) are persons trained to portray a patient with a particular presentation and can be used for demonstration, formative and summative evaluation (Miller, 1993). SP demonstration may be particularly useful when the subject area is difficult or uncomfortable to learn from real patients, as is the case with the Pap test. SPs can be trained to give immediate feedback to the student during the examination or interview (Robertson, 1999).

The use of SPs in the teaching of gynaecological examinations has advantages over other methods of instruction, such as lectures, videos, demonstration and practice on plastic models or patients in outpatient clinics and general practice. These include (Abraham, 1995; O'Connor, 1999):

- focus on normal anatomy in a non-threatening, less time-pressured learning environment;
- increased realism;
- increased focus on communication skills and the doctor-patient relationship;
- immediate feedback from an experienced patient;
- standardisation of the learning experience;

- convenience of scheduling; and
- limitation of ethical problems with the use of real patients.

The students themselves are aware of these advantages, for, as one noted, this [is] a difficult subject to find opportunity to learn from and discuss with patients in the clinical setting.

Despite the extensive use of these programs in North America and their more recent development in Australia, there has been very limited evaluation that has been published. Kleinman demonstrated that there was no significant difference in technical skills between medical students trained to perform pelvic examinations by laywomen (acting as teachers and patients) and those who had been trained by doctors (as teachers with a laywoman serving as a patient) (N = 81) (Kleinman, 1996). However, the laywoman-trained students demonstrated significantly better *interpersonal* skills than did the doctor-trained students (p = .01). Although the majority of CTA programs are aimed at improving communication skills, there is a lack of published evidence both here and overseas of the efficacy of the programs in achieving this aim.

Until recently, only three of Australia's ten medical schools used Gynaecological Teaching Associate programs. A Clinical Teaching Associates in Gynaecology program (CTA) to teach the well woman examination was established in 1996 by the Department of Obstetrics and Gynaecology at the University of Queensland with the financial support of the Queensland Cancer Fund (O'Connor, 1999). It is currently taught in the second year of the graduate MBBS Program. A year later researchers from the Department of General Practice, University of Melbourne began to work with PapScreen Victoria to devise educational programs to improve the skills and knowledge of general practitioners in the area of cervical screening. A review of the literature reinforced the belief that Victorian women were likely to benefit if medical students, as well as practicing doctors, had access to high quality training in cervical screening such as that provided by a clinical teaching associate program (Hegarty and Gunn, 2000). The CTA program funded by PapScreen Victoria also includes tutorials to teach sensitive breast examination skills to all third year medical students at Melbourne and Monash Universities. This paper will focus on the Well Woman Check tutorials for fifth year medical students at the University of Melbourne to enable illustration of issues for a recently established program in an Australian setting. Staff involved with CTA programs overseas will gain current insights into contemporary issues around development and evaluation of CTA programs.

THE CTA PROGRAM IN VICTORIA

The CTA program in Victoria was developed in accordance with the published literature to include:

- a clearly identified coordinator–the CTA program built on, and drew upon the expertise in medical education and use of simulated patients developed within the Department of General Practice over the past decade;
- ongoing recruitment strategies;
- clear role description for CTAs;
- a comprehensive training program;
- on-going support; and
- sound medical education principles.

A CTA program is labor intensive. It is essential that a suitably qualified medical educator coordinate the program to maintain quality assurance, assist in recruitment, oversee evaluation, training of CTAs, and staff development and ensure sustainability. Administrative assistance is required to organize recruitment campaigns, arrange timetables and payment, process evaluation forms and assist with report writing.

A multidisciplinary reference group was formed with broad representation. This reference group[1] has played an important role in facilitating the first steps of the program by ensuring integration into the existing curriculum, and identifying additional educational opportunities.

Recruitment of CTAs

Recruitment of women is a key step towards a successful program. CTAs are required to demonstrate the sensitivity and perspective of a woman presenting for a well woman check, and to develop refined and specialized skills in pelvic examination technique and instruction, specialized knowledge of female pelvic anatomy, excellent interpersonal skills, and non-membership of the medical profession (Kretzschmar, 1978). The aim is to recruit women who already possess, or who can be trained in these qualities. In addition to the above, selection criteria for CTAs were adapted from the University of Queensland criteria (O'Connor, 1999) and included:

- a strong commitment to improving the well-being of women and their treatment within the health care system;
- motivation and enthusiasm;
- good communication skills;
- good health, including normal breasts and pelvic anatomy;
- being comfortable with own body and how it works;
- being intelligent, mature and responsible; and
- being available to work when required.

Initially, women were recruited through short advertisements in local newspapers, notices in hospital and community health care clinics, and through various women's networks. Quite specific advertisements were more successful. The largest single recruitment source was through the Life Models Association, which also had the advantage of reaching women of broad age ranges and physical characteristics.

On expressing interest in joining the program, women are sent a brief information pack outlining the purpose and structure of the program. They are invited to an orientation session, during which the CTA program aims and structure, and the roles of the CTAs are explained. An outline of the Well Woman Check, barriers to screening, an overview of the traditional methods of training in this area and the benefits of a CTA program, both to the students themselves and to their future patients, are also covered in the orientation. Finally their terms and conditions of employment are detailed. The women are advised that they can discontinue their involvement at any stage, that they will be placed on a three-month probation period to ascertain their suitability to the program and the program for them, that the program will not offer the CTA medical care, and that women should attend their own practitioner for a check before and during the program.

Training

Women who decide to continue with the program undertake a series of training workshops (see Box 1). CTAs need a clear understanding of the aims and philosophy underpinning the program, appreciate the educational stages of students and doctors they will be working with, and being comfortable in the various tasks. They need to become skilled in the content and process of the various components of a well woman check, to be able to provide specific, sensitive and constructive feedback and to develop team skills and cohesiveness. The training also aims to achieve standardization so that learners are ensured of equivalent training experiences.

CTAs need to be trained in different tasks including: session leader, introduction leader, demonstration doctor, patient and buddy (see Box 2). The Well Woman Check tutorials for all fifth year medical students are run by the CTAs independently according to the format designed by the Program medical education staff. This direct interaction between CTAs and students is one of the strengths of the program.

CTAs begin to be rostered on to work after the first training session, initially only in roles that they are skilled and comfortable in, and with the ongoing support, guidance and supervision of more experienced CTAs. Subsequent training sessions have been held every 6 weeks in the first year. These have the purpose of establishing and enhancing a group identity and CTA relationships, provide a forum for identifying and dealing with any issues that arise, and provide specific ongoing training in multiple skills areas.

BOX 1. CTA Training

Module 1

The CTA tutorial

 Outline

 Expectations for CTAs and students

 Student evaluation

The breast examination

 Anatomy and physiology

 Breast changes

 Breast examination techniques–theory

Female genitalia and reproductive organs

 Anatomy and physiology

 Examination theory

Instruments used in a Pap test

Communication skills

 Barriers to screening

 Language and informed consent

Live demonstration of a best practice well-woman examination

Infection control

 Correct glove technique

Equipment

Undertaking the well-woman check on each other under supervision, support and guidance

---

Module 2: Being a Buddy

Role and responsibilities of Buddy CTA

When and how to intervene

What to do if you (or the student) can't find the cervix

Providing feedback to students

Module 3: The Demonstration Doctor and Debriefing

Role and responsibilities of demonstration doctor

Debriefing with students and each other

Professional relationships

Dealing with abnormalities

How to call a stop/pause

Module 4: A Learner-Centred Approach

Evaluation results

Culture and its impact on the tutorial/consultation

Maslow's Hierarchy (of learning needs)

BOX 2. CTA Session Format

Each tutorial involves four students and four CTAs. Each session runs for just under 2 1/2 hours and consists of introduction, demonstration, role-play in pairs and debriefing.

Introduction

The first half-hour is given to the introduction. This involves introducing the CTAs to the students, reviewing student and CTA expectations for the tutorial, reminding the students of the components of a Well Woman Check, including the importance of good communication, and addressing student anxiety. (Prior to the CTA tutorial, the students have been able to access detailed information about the Well Woman Check.) The equipment is discussed, and the students are encouraged to handle a speculum and become familiar and comfortable with it.

Demonstration

The next half-hour involves a demonstration of a 'best-practice' well woman consultation. Two CTAs demonstrate the well woman check. The entire consultation is role-played so the students can observe a full well woman check before undertaking a supervised examination themselves.

Role play in pairs

Students and CTAs pair up for the major learning component of the session. Over the next hour, the CTAs guide the students through the well woman check. Each student gets the opportunity to perform the consultation with immediate feedback, in addition to viewing one other student in the same clinic room perform the check. Two CTAs work in partnership, one guiding the student, giving feedback from an instructor's perspective and supporting the CTA being examined (the Buddy CTA), while the other is examined and offers feedback from the patient perspective. The CTAs then change roles and the next student has the opportunity to conduct the examination.

Debriefing

CTAs and students are encouraged to talk about the afternoon's activities and share their experiences (successes and difficulties). After the students leave, the CTAs have their own debriefing session in which they are encouraged to identify any issues they encountered, either personally or with their student.

Evaluation

Evaluation data has been collected from the programs at the Universities of Queensland and Melbourne, and this paper reports on both sets of data.

The University of Queensland CTA program asked the students (N = 275) about their expectations and concerns before taking part in a CTA session. The main expectations were to improve their communication skills (20%), understand women's fears (9%), learn a 'sensitive' approach (6%), and overcome their own embarrassment (5.5%). The most significant fear was that of hurting the woman during the examination (57%), followed by a feeling of embarrassment themselves (17%), causing anxiety or embarrassing for the CTA (14%), and concern that they might do 'something wrong' (13%). After the sessions the students were asked for open comments on positive and negative aspects of the session (Table 1).

At The University of Melbourne, an evaluation questionnaire was provided to each student after they had participated in a CTA tutorial. Students were required to rate their level of comfort before, during and after the session and to comment on how the nature of the subject matter, the learning environment and the CTA affected this level. Comments on the contribution of the CTA session towards development of practical and communication skills were also sought. Finally, students were offered the opportunity to comment on any positive or negative aspects of their session, or the program in general, and to provide suggestions for improvement. The overall response rate was 91% (N = 67). Responses to the questions are summarized below.

The intimate nature of learning to perform a sensitive examination can be a confronting experience for many students and this has potential to impede learning. Figure 1 shows self-reported ratings of comfort before, during, and after the CTA session. Students reported increasing comfort levels over the course of the session. The proportion of students who rated their level of comfort between 1 and 4 increased from 45 percent before the session to almost 60 percent during the session, and to over 80 percent after the session, as indicated by students' responses to qualitative questions:

> The tutors were quite relaxed about it, which made it much easier for us.

> The CTA was very professional and that in itself made it much easier for us.

> Very helpful. Felt like I could ask them anything.

> Good to do the first one on a friendly, understanding subject, where mistakes can be addressed openly, unlike in the clinical situation.

The role of the CTA in creating a non-threatening environment conducive to learning was acknowledged and valued by students. There were few negative aspects of the program, in general concerning the opportunity for all stu-

TABLE 1. Student Comments on CTA Session (N = 275)

CTAs were friendly, helpful and supportive	55%
Session practical and 'real'	36%
Relaxed learning environment	27%
Improved communication skills	24%
Increased confidence with well woman check	22%

FIGURE 1. Self-reported ratings of comfort level before, during and after session.

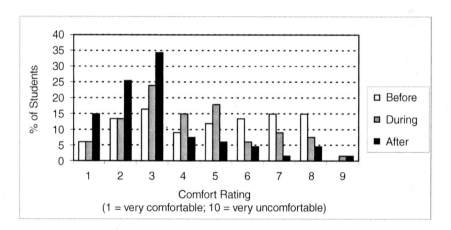

dents to have the tutorial early in their training, and providing for further opportunities to practice.

Students were particularly appreciative of the opportunity to get feedback from a patient's perspective:

> CTAs very knowledgeable. Positive feedback before negative/constructive comments was a fantastic (and unusual!) experience.

> Good to practice on a real person and get feedback. This is impossible to get from a patient without embarrassing all involved.

> Very valuable–especially feedback.

Students reported an increased awareness of communication issues during sensitive examinations. In particular the importance of using appropriate verbal and non-verbal communication was highlighted.

> Really made me think about what comes out of my mouth and how simple words can be misconstrued.

> CTA reinforced how important it was to keep communicating with the patient during the examination.

> It made me realise the importance of explaining every step of the examination to the patient.

ISSUES IN THE ESTABLISHMENT OF A CTA PROGRAM

Relationships Between CTAs

CTAs work in very intimate ways with each other–physically and emotionally–and depend on each other to protect their well-being. They need to develop professional relationships which allow this intimacy, but also have clear and mutually recognized boundaries. There are similarities with the professional nature of the doctor-patient relationship, but made more complex by the bilateral nature of the intimacy. Stressing the professional nature of the interactions can counterbalance this intimacy. This is done by formalizing and providing structure to the different aspects of the relationship, and ensuring that contact and follow up outside the tutorial structure is through the CTA coordinator.

Cultural Diversity

Although there is some ethnic diversity among the current pool of CTAs, this does not reflect the breadth of diversity of the wider community nor adequately represent under-screened communities. Ideally, the pool should include representatives of these under-screened groups such as older women and those from Aboriginal and Non-English Speaking backgrounds, and thus reinforce the importance of encouraging all women to participate in screening.

The background of the students also needs to be considered in these potentially very confronting tutorials. As a group, the students in the graduate medical course at the University of Queensland are older and tend to have more world experience than the predominantly undergraduate students at the University of Melbourne. Of the first year intake into the medical course at the

University of Melbourne, 30.5% are International students, predominantly from Southeast Asia, who may bring their own attitudes towards such issues as respect for teachers, demonstration of anxiety or uncertainty, assertive women, sexually confident women, physical contact and comfort with nakedness which impact on their approach to the tutorial. An individual's past experiences, beliefs, comfort and attitudes are more important than broad group generalizations, but the impact of culture should not be underestimated. For this reason, one of the training sessions for the CTAs specifically focuses on the student, to encourage the CTAs to take a learner-centred approach.

Comfort and Self-Esteem

As well as a narrow ethnic diversity, women who become CTAs are not representative of the broader community in other aspects. Many women find the components of the well woman examination so embarrassing, uncomfortable or degrading that they do not present for biannual checks; CTAs are prepared to be examined up to twice per week. They come from all walks of life, yet share a comfort and knowledge of their own bodies and a sense of personal empowerment that they can make a difference to the health care provided to women. Studies elsewhere have indicated a small, steady increase in self-esteem in GTAs/CTAs (Beckmann, 1988). A core objective of the training is that the students become more skilled in identifying and appropriately dealing with patients' discomfort, and the training needs to be clear that most women will not be as comfortable, nor as assertive as the CTAs.

Power and Authority

The women in the CTA program act as both patient and teacher. This latter role represents a significant shift in the power balance of the environment in which medical students and doctors usually learn to undertake Pap tests (and, indeed, most aspects of the physical examination). Patients in outpatient clinics, general practice or as inpatients are often cast in a dependent role, by the nature of their circumstances, which limits their power in interactions with students. Certainly anaesthetized patients and pelvic models are passive in the extreme, and whatever skills students learn from examining them may have little bearing on undertaking a real well woman check. The communication and sensitivity required before, during and after an intimate examination is not easily learnt in these environments.

Ethical Considerations

The use of standardized patients in the training of medical students overcomes the ethical concerns of using real patients who are already vulnerable and dependent by the nature of their illness (Robertson, 1999). There are genuine concerns about such issues as informed and free consent, and the modeling of inappropriate doctor-patient relationships and power imbalances when real patients participate in the training of future doctors.

However, the use of CTAs raises particular ethical issues itself. A program such as that described in this paper needs to make CTA safety and comfort a prime objective, but this may sometimes come into conflict with the training needs of the learners. Women who are employed as CTAs have a strong focus on improving the skills of the medical students, even putting up with considerable discomfort–both physical and emotional–because the students have to learn. CTAs need to be continuously encouraged and supported to make clear their discomfort, and given training in how to do so.

While immediate feedback and debriefing is a crucial part of the tutorial, it may only be afterwards, on reflection, that a CTA's sense of disquiet develops into a stronger belief of impropriety (this is often the case in real-life interactions, as well). Although this has been a rare occurrence in this program, CTAs need to be able to contact the program coordinator at any time after a tutorial to discuss any issues which are troubling them, and a mechanism must be established for following this up with the students involved, and those responsible for their training. It is important that CTAs know that such follow up will occur.

CTAs are few in number. Currently 14 women participate in the University of Melbourne program. A balance needs to be achieved between providing enough work to maintain interest, involvement and skills and having enough CTAs to cover all needs and eventualities (such as menstruation).

Care also has to be taken to respect privacy of the CTAs, some of whom may choose not to disclose the nature of their work to family and friends. Care is not only taken with contact from program staff, but the importance of confidentiality is stressed to students in the introduction.

Students also need to have their privacy respected. CTAs are in a unique position to observe student behaviour from the lay perspective. Experienced CTAs become skilled at identifying students with special needs, especially those who have poor or very limited communication skills. CTAs in this intimate situation are able to detect those students who are displaying negative attitudes towards women and who are unable to deal with the sensitive nature of the examination. In this situation the CTA addresses the problem with the student and the need to feedback to the program coordinator. The coordinator will then refer the student on to a designated clinician for assistance and support.

CONCLUSION

Providing an intensive learning experience such as described in this paper requires committed funding. The Victorian program has been created by program funding from PapScreen Victoria, but other funding is required if the program is to secure a future. Program directors need to strike a balance between program expansion and sustainability.

Development and implementation of a CTA program at The University of Melbourne is the first step towards ensuring that every medical graduate in the state has at least one opportunity to experience what it is like to perform an intimate examination in a woman-centred way. These are early days for the Victorian program and yet we have achieved so much. A dedicated group of women form the core of the CTA program. We have managed to provide high quality training and support to these women and have learnt much from them in return. The preliminary evaluation presented here demonstrates just how much medical students appreciate the opportunity to practice an intimate examination like the Pap test in a supportive and educative environment.

A program such as this requires comprehensive and in-depth evaluation using quantitative and qualitative methods to capture the experience of students, CTAs and the program coordinators. The program can also be offered as a package to other medical schools and to practicing clinicians, preferably in coalition with existing continuing medical education providers. Ideally, the cohort of medical students who have undertaken such training should be followed up in future years to assess the long-term impact of the program.

AUTHORS NOTE

The authors would like to acknowledge the invaluable contributions of the staff of PapScreen Victoria, the Faculty Education Unit of the Faculty of Medicine, University of Melbourne and the members of the Reference Group. They would like to thank Jacinta Lee and Cate Nagle for all their work in the administration and evaluation of the program, and the students for their considered feedback. Finally they would like to acknowledge the skills and dedication of all the CTAs, and the CTA coordinators: Helen Lockhart and Debbie Anderson (Qld) and Kerrilie Rice (Vic).

NOTE

1. The reference group consisted of representatives from the AntiCancer Council; Victorian Cytology Service; the Royal Australian College of General Practitioners Training Program; General Practice Divisions Victoria; Family Planning Victoria; The Faculty Education Unit of the Faculty of Medicine, University of Melbourne; The Royal Women's Hospital; Monash University's Faculty of Medicine and Nurse Practitioners.

REFERENCES

Abraham, S. (1995). Vaginal and speculum examination in medical curricula. *Australian and New Zealand Journal of Obstetrics and Gynaecology* 35, 56-60.

Alexander, K., McCullough, J. (1981). Women's preferences for gynecological examiners: sex versus role. *Women & Health* 6, 123-134.

Beckmann, C.R.B., Barzansky, B.M., Sharf, B.F., Meyers, K. (1988). Training gynaecological teaching associates. *Medical Education* 22, 124-131.

Beckmann, C.R.B., Meyers, K. (1988). Mental and physical effects of being a gynecologic teaching associate. *The Journal of Reproductive Medicine* 23, 22-24.

Cockburn, J., White, V.M., Hirst, S., Hill, D. (1992). Barriers to cervical screening in older women. *Australian Family Physician* 21, 973-978.

Evans, B., Stanley, R.O., et al. (1992). Measuring medical students' communication skills: development and evaluation of an interview rating scale. *Psychology and Health* 6, 213-225.

Fernbach, M. (1999). Barriers to Cervical Screening. Melbourne, PapScreen Victoria, Centre for Behavioural Research in Cancer.

Goertzen, J., Steward, M., Weston, W. (1995). Effective teaching behaviours of rural family medicine preceptors. *Canadian Medical Association* 153(2, July 15), 161-168.

Gridley, H., Moore, S., Higgins, J., Johnson, K. (1998). Improving women's health care: The experiences of women patients and general practitioners in the western region of Melbourne. *Australian Journal of Primary Health–Interchange* 4(3), 119-133.

Hegarty, K., Gunn, J. (2000). Towards Sensitive Pap Examinations by Medical Practitioners. Melbourne, Department of General Practice & Public Health, University of Melbourne.

Hill, D., Gardner, G., Rassaby, J. (1985). Factors predisposing women to take precautions against breast and cervix cancer. *Journal of Applied Social Psychology* 15, 59-79.

Kann, P.E., Lane, D.S. (1998). Breast cancer screening knowledge and skills of students upon entering and exiting a medical school. *Academic Medicine* 73(8), 904-906.

Kleinman, D.E., Hage, M.L., Hoole, A.J., Kowlowitz, V. (1996). Pelvic examination instruction and experience: A comparison of laywoman-trained and physician-trained students. *Academic Medicine* 71(11), 1239-1243.

Kretzschmar, R.M. (1978). Evolution of the gynecology teaching associate: An education specialist. *American Journal of Obstetrics and Gynecology* 131, 367-373.

Lang, F. (1990). Resident behaviours during observed pelvic examinations. *Family Medicine* 22(2), 153-155.

Lewis, D., Mitchell, H. (1994). An evaluation of cervical screening in general practice. *Medical Journal Australia* 160, 628-632.

Lurie, N., Margolis, K., McGovern, P.G., Mink, P. (1998). Physician self-report of comfort and skill in providing preventive care to patients of the opposite sex. *Archives of Family Medicine* 7(2, Mar-Apr), 134-137.

Miller, G.E. (1993). Conference summary. *Academic Medicine* 68, 471-474.

Moore, S., Gridley, H., Taylor, K., Johnson, K. (2000). Women's views about intimate examinations and sexually inappropriate practices by their general practitioners. *Psychology and Health* 15, 71-84.

National Health and Medical Research Council (1997). Promoting the health of Australians-case studies of achievements in improving the health of the population. Canberra.

O'Connor, V. (1999). Clinical teaching associates in gynaecology. Queensland, The University of QLD, QLD Cancer Fund.

Petravage, J.B., Reynolds, L.J., Gardner, H.J., Reading, J.C. (1979). Attitudes of women towards the gynecologic examination. *Journal of Family Practice* 9, 1039-1045.

Robertson, K. (1999). It really felt real: The introduction of simulated patients to the communication skills course for third year medical students at the University of Melbourne. *Faculty of Education.* The University of Melbourne.

Shelley, J., Irwig, L., Simpson, J.M., Macaskill, P. (1991). Evaluation of a mass media-led campaign to increase pap smear screening. *Health Education Research* 6, 267-277.

Straton, J. (1994). Recruiting for cervical screening: A review of the literature. Western Australia, Dept. of Public Health, The University of Western Australia.

Taylor, D.M. (1997). Undergraduate procedural skills training in Victoria: Is it adequate? *Medical Journal of Australia* 166(5), 251-254.

Ward, J., Harding, N., Sanson-Fisher, R. (1997). Trainees' interactional skills when performing Pap smears. *Australian Family Physician* 26(2), 147-151.

Gender and the Medical Curriculum:
A Rural Case Study

Jo Wainer, MA

SUMMARY. In Australia, half the medical students are women. There is increasing evidence that women engage with medicine differently from men, and medical workforce planners are being required to consider the implications of this change, particularly in areas of medical need. Between 1996-2001, the Australian government provided funding for teaching about issues for female rural doctors to encourage female students to consider rural medical practice. This was extended to include teaching about gender issues for doctors. Introducing this teaching has required building credibility for the topic among funders, faculty and students, training tutors, and meeting the need of students for an intellectual framework within which to think about gender and medicine. Teaching about gender requires conscious leadership by senior academic

Jo Wainer is Social Scientist and Senior Lecturer, Monash University Faculty of Medicine, Nursing and Health Sciences.

Address correspondence to: Jo Wainer, School of Rural Health, Box 64, Monash University, VIC 3800, Australia (E-mail: Jo.Wainer@med.monash.edu.au).

This work was made possible by the cooperation and dedication of rural doctors who first learnt, and then taught with skilled commitment, the curriculum as honorary staff of the University. Our greatest teachers were our students, who chose to take the risk and attend tutorials on gender issues for rural doctors.

This curriculum development work was funded by the Rural Undergraduate Support and Coordination Program of the Commonwealth Government's Department of Health and Ageing.

[Haworth co-indexing entry note]: "Gender and the Medical Curriculum: A Rural Case Study." Wainer, Jo. Co-published simultaneously in *Women & Health* (The Haworth Medical Press, an imprint of The Haworth Press, Inc.) Vol. 37, No. 4, 2003, pp. 67-87; and: *Teaching Gender, Teaching Women's Health: Case Studies in Medical and Health Science Education* (ed: Lenore Manderson) The Haworth Medical Press, an imprint of The Haworth Press, Inc., 2003, pp. 67-87. Single or multiple copies of this article are available for a fee from The Haworth Document Delivery Service [1-800-HAWORTH, 9:00 a.m. - 5:00 p.m. (EST). E-mail address: docdelivery@haworthpress.com].

women. This paper describes an initiative in the rural curriculum for medical students. *[Article copies available for a fee from The Haworth Document Delivery Service: 1-800-HAWORTH. E-mail address: <docdelivery@ haworthpress.com> Website: <http://www.HaworthPress.com> © 2003 by The Haworth Press, Inc. All rights reserved.]*

KEYWORDS. Gender and medicine, teaching gender, medical curriculum, rural medical curriculum

At all stages this process should be needs-driven, evidence-based, learner-centred, and outcome-measured.

Rourke and Strasser (1996:468)

Monash University, in Melbourne, Australia, teaches a curriculum unit on Gender Issues for Rural Doctors to undergraduate medical students. The unit focuses on gender within medicine, including the construction of medical knowledge, professional structures, reward systems, and sustainable ways women and men have found to work as rural doctors. Development of the unit was funded by the Commonwealth Government of Australia as part of a long-term, vertically-integrated strategy to attract and retain doctors in rural medical practice.

Three factors underpinned the development of the curriculum unit. The first was the increase in female medical students, combined with increasing evidence about the different ways women and men interact with their medical careers. The second was the long-standing worldwide shortage of doctors working in rural and remote practice, including Australia. The third was a political imperative to improve health services to rural and remote Australians. The seemingly simple task of developing and teaching a curriculum unit about issues for female rural doctors turned out to be both complex and challenging.

FACILITATIVE ENVIRONMENT

Women and Men in Medicine

The maldistribution of doctors has been identified as an important equity and workforce issue in many countries (Makin 1998), confounded by the increasing presence of women, and the different ways female and male doctors contribute to medicine. Doctors are underrepresented in rural and impoverished areas, and female doctors are less likely to go into rural practice than their male colleagues (Wainer, Carson & Strasser 2000). Levitt and McEwin (2001) have pointed out that increasing female participation in the medical workforce, combined with the different work characteristics of male and female doctors, is likely to have a substantial impact on the future supply and distribution of medical practitioners. Australian data demonstrate that female doctors tend to chose general (family) practice, and work part-time in capital cities or major urban areas. Women are also likely to leave medicine or practice at quite low activity levels for a period of time during their careers (Australian Medical Workforce Advisory Committee 1998). On average they work fewer hours over a lifetime than male doctors (Australian Medical Workforce Advisory Committee & Australian Institute of Health and Welfare 1996).

While doctors have a shared body of knowledge, core competencies and professional ethos, there are different preferred working styles that can be identified as favoured by women and men (Turner, Tippett & Raphael 1994; Hojat, Gonnella & Xu 1995; Moodley, Barnes & de Villiers 1999; Wainer 2001). An Australian study (Redman, Saltman et al. 1994) found that female doctors are more influenced than men in their choice of speciality by the need for "the opportunity for holistic care." Their availability for clinical practice is strongly influenced by their status as mothers (Wainer 2001). Britt et al. (1995, 1999) found that by comparison with males, female family doctors tend to have longer consultations, manage significantly higher numbers of problems per encounter, see a higher percentage of younger patients and new patients, and manage depression more often. Patients are much less likely to present to male doctors with issues of interpersonal violence or sexual assault (Wainer 1998). In general, female doctors value psychosocial aspects of health more than men do, and tend to operate more strongly from a biopsychosocial rather than biomedical paradigm. These different priorities are reflected in different styles of practice (Australian Medical Workforce Advisory Committee 1998) and combine with different expectations from patients (Rogers 1995; Bundrock 1996; Brown, Young & Byles 1997). Thus, while western medicine has always been practiced by men and there has been an unacknowledged convergence between "medicine" and "male-practiced medicine," the presence of women in sufficient numbers has raised the possibility that there is a way to practice medicine that reflects the priorities and values of female doctors.

Rural Workforce

The estimated shortage of rural doctors (1,000 doctors) in Australia includes an even greater shortage of female rural doctors. Less than a quarter of the rural medical workforce are women (Strasser et al. 1997), although women comprise 27% of medical practitioners and half of all graduating medical students. It is essential to understand how young women relate to their profession if they are to be attracted into rural practice. Several papers (Thompson 1997; Carson & Stringer 1998; Wainer 1998) have analysed the evidence for an emerging cultural change within the rural medical workforce, and Tolhurst et al. (1997) have drawn out some of the tensions experienced by female rural doctors. In general, female students and doctors considering rural practice have had to adapt to a male culture in medicine, and the unquestioned masculinity of rural environments. Making this explicit and articulating some consequences and solutions was an important feature of the development of the gender curriculum.

DEVELOPMENT OF THE CURRICULUM

Development of the curriculum was funded by the Rural Undergraduate Support and Coordination (RUSC) program, part of the General Practice Branch of the Commonwealth Department of Health and Aged Care. RUSC is funded to implement long-term strategic programs to increase the number of rural doctors. These include facilitating rural students into medical courses, increasing medical teaching in rural areas, establishing a rural club at each medical faculty, providing scholarships for students from rural backgrounds and for students to spend time in rural and remote areas, holding annual meetings of rural clubs and rural medical academics, and as a Project of National Significance, teaching about gender issues for rural doctors.

The first academic Undergraduate Rural Curriculum Conference in 1994 concluded that there was a primary need for greater understanding by medical schools of the ethos and culture of rural areas (Hanemaaijer 1995). The introduction of teaching about gendered medicine in the rural curriculum refines that objective to focus on the need for greater understanding of the interaction between the ethos and culture of rural areas, and their intersection with the ethos and culture of women and men as medical practitioners.

The development of a curriculum unit that expands existing norms needs to be presented in a form that can be advocated and supported in a compelling way (Schei 1996). Rourke and Strasser were talking about the introduction of a rural curriculum when they determined: "At all stages this process should be needs-driven, evidence-based, learner-centred, and outcome-measured" (Rourke and Strasser 1996:468). Their comments apply equally to the introduction of curriculum on gender issues in medical practice.

The initial aims of the curriculum development project were to:

- Encourage female family doctors to work in rural practice by exposing medical students to the professional and personal strategies for success and well-being developed by women already practising in rural general practice.

- Expand understanding of the issues for women in rural general practice that increase or decrease their probability of working in rural areas.
- Begin to develop proposals for change that will increase the attraction of rural practice for women.

This was later expanded to include the development of a gender vocabulary and gender competency in professional interactions.

The curriculum was initially about women and rural medical practice. When it became clear that this held little interest for male students, it was expanded to encompass gender issues for rural doctors. The primary intention of the new curriculum was to provide a framework for students to explore the experience of being women and men in medicine, and to apply that to rural practice. In addition, female rural family doctors were trained to teach the unit, providing role models so that female students were assisted to see themselves as potential rural doctors. The framework needed to be consistent with that developed by the RUSC Undergraduate Rural Curriculum Conference (Hanemaaijer 1995). Curriculum is to be based on adult-learning principles incorporating problem-based and experiential learning, as these most accurately reflect learning in rural practice. Course materials are to be based on the learner's "need to know" and stage of development, self-directed, and based on real life cases. Rural-based personnel should be used in educational planning and teaching of rural practice, and recognised and supported by medical school faculty. The relative lack of visibility of women as teachers of medicine compounded the importance of drawing on the expertise of female rural practitioners in developing and teaching this curriculum.

Students

The curriculum framework and development of teaching materials began in 1996 with a literature review that identified existing work on how female medical students and doctors relate to medicine. A small proportion of this work included the rural medical experience (Rourke et al. 1996; Tolhurst et al. 1997). This was followed by discussions with female rural medical students from Monash University and The University of Melbourne, and a survey of first and third year students at Monash University to ensure the contemporary relevance of the curriculum.

Second year students identified concerns about sexism in rural environments, competence in women's health in anticipation that they would be called upon to provide that, concerns about how they would manage to have a family and be a country doctor, and whether as women they would attract the same respect as that accorded male doctors. They expressed a need to work with female rural doctors if possible as "we have been given the impression that there

are no women in rural practice because it is too hard." They suggested a
two-day workshop at each of years 2, 4 and 5. Fourth year students fresh from
exposure to the culture of rural hospitals were confused and upset about the
discontinuity of their view of themselves as fully valued "doctors-in-training"
and the put-down comments made by some of their teachers. Fifth year students outlined a number of gender issues that had been apparent during rural
rotations, including the importance of seeing female rural doctors at work, the
importance of having a partner, balancing patient demand for women's health
with other areas of practice, and the extended nature of rural practice.

A questionnaire was developed on the basis of issues raised by this consultation and the survey was carried out by student members of the Rural Practice
Association at Monash University. One hundred and seventy-two (172) medical students of a student body of 291 completed the questionnaire. One hundred and eight (108) female and 58 male students responded; six students did
not specify their sex. Seventy-seven percent said they had considered how they
might combine family and professional life, with more females (81%) than
male students (69%) likely to have thought about it. A majority felt that this
was likely to be more difficult in rural areas, and female students were more
aware of this than the male students (62% compared with 53%). Asked
whether they wanted an opportunity to discuss these issues, 73% of students
said yes (81% female, 59% male), most in an informal setting. Nineteen percent of the students thought sexism in rural communities was different from
their experience in urban areas and 13% gave examples of this difference.
Twenty-eight percent of those who completed the questionnaire had at least
one year living in rural or remote areas while still at school, reflecting the pref-
erential selection of rural origin students into medicine at Monash. Finally, the
students were asked whether gender was an issue for them. Seventeen percent
said it was while a further nine percent made some written comment in response to this question. More female than male students said it was an issue for
them (21% compared with 12%). These discussions provided some content
and sequencing advice for the curriculum, and assurance that teaching about
gender issues was meeting an identified learning need.

FRAMEWORK

Discussion with faculty responsible for undergraduate rural teaching se-
cured their agreement to include this topic in second year and sixth year, although there was some scepticism in the general faculty committees. The
Professor of Rural Health has control of the rural curriculum, and it took his
authorisation, with the support of a senior female rural medical academic, to
overcome the hesitancy.

The Specific Objectives for Rural General Practice Education at Monash University guide the whole of the rural general practice teaching. They were amended to include an objective: "To increase students' understanding of issues which specifically relate to women doctors in rural areas including personal, professional and family issues." The preceptor manual for Monash University and the University of Melbourne Rural General Practitioner Teacher Training was amended to include a case in which gender issues influenced the outcome of the management. The preceptors are asked to consider examples of gender issues they have experienced or observed in their practice and how this could contribute to achieving this objective.

Second year students undertake a compulsory attachment in rural health. At the pre-briefing, they are asked to observe and take notes on a health care event in which the sex of the participants affected the process or the outcome. Students are also instructed to observe and take notes on personal and professional aspects of rural medical practice for women and bring them to the debriefing when they return. They are not assessed on this task. Second year students based at the rural town of Traralgon also take part in a one hour tutorial on gender issues in medicine.

Sixth year students at Monash University spend two weeks in a rural general practice. They are encouraged to observe the effects of gender on the work and family experiences of family doctors. These students also complete a compulsory three week term in a rural hospital and are offered a one hour tutorial on Gender Issues for Rural Doctors for each of the three weeks. The objective of the teaching is to provide the students with a critical framework within which to think about how sex and gender influence the experience of rural medical practice and medicine in general. A secondary objective is to provide role models for female students who are interested in rural medicine.

TEACHING THE CURRICULUM

General Practice Rotation

Final year students undertake two weeks with a rural family doctor and are assessed on their learning. This assessment includes two short essays and the students can choose an objective of rural general practice learning to write about. Many write about gender, and on the whole, the essays are thoughtful and observant. Female students who work with female rural doctors reflect on how the roles of female and rural doctor can be made to work. Male and female students observe how patients present differently to doctors of each sex and the implications this has for professional practice. A male student observed "Many patients feel that female doctors are more caring and sensitive than their male colleagues," and that in a rural environment without allied health support, this resulted in female doctors being sought out by patients for counselling and emotional support.

The students are aware of how highly valued female rural doctors are, as the following comments illustrate:

> Female doctors are rare commodities in rural areas . . . and the need for female doctors is paramount.
>
> She believes that her return to a medical career after having her family would not have been possible if she had remained living in a large city. The supportive rural community, and close collaboration with other doctors in the area and . . . the confidence and encouragement given by the local community . . . have meant that she had the courage to persevere and establish a practice.

The students observed that this valuing resulted in waiting lists ("the women doctors were always booked weeks in advance") and pressure to provide professional services, but it also provided opportunities to structure rural medicine to suit the doctor's need for time for self and family. They are also aware of the extended role of rural medicine and the professional challenges this provides, and are attracted to this:

> She saw the move to rural practice as a great challenge, where she would be provided with a huge spectrum of medical, social and psychological issues, which she would have the freedom to tackle as she saw fit.

Both students and female doctors comment on how being female impacts on rural medicine. One doctor is quoted as saying "when I first started in country practice, there was very little conversation and interaction between me and my male colleagues. It was as though I had X chromosome written all over me. No one would talk to me." This doctor noted that she was now much more assertive and confident, especially in her practical skills, since undertaking rural practice.

On their rural attachment, the students observed that female rural family doctors generally do Pap smears, gynaecology and counselling, and that they are often part-time or regarded as part-time. Female final year students sometimes expressed anger that they may be expected to do this "limited" clinical practice rather than the more general spectrum of care that they saw the male rural doctors practice and that they are also trained to do. The female students also occasionally reported lack of job satisfaction for female family doctors and they equated this to the "limited" care they practice.

Students take part in a seminar on their return from their rural family practice attachment. The seminars are led by a senior female academic rural doctor who explores gender issues as part of the discussion. She found that students do not volunteer their observations about gender issues unless specifically invited to do so. Once the topic had been introduced, however, students of both sexes appreciated the opportunity to discuss gender issues. Final year students are more aware of these issues than the younger students.

Hospital Rotation

Final year students also spend a compulsory three week rotation in a rural hospital. The gender curriculum is taught in weekly tutorials. There are eight students per rotation at one hospital, four at the second hospital and two at the third. The tutorials vary from group to group, and one of the main factors is the balance of male and female students in the group. In groups comprised of all or predominantly male students who are not interested in rural practice, the students have difficulty relating to the subject matter. Gender is not self-evident as an issue for the dominant culture. In groups that have a more even sex ratio, the students are quick to see the relevance of the topics raised.

Learner-centred teaching. *Tutorials were developed to reflect the knowledge and experience the students brought with them. This was enhanced toward the end of the year by the opportunity to reflect on gender in rural practice from their general practice rotation.* The topics of the tutorials varied with the interest of the student group, and included clinical presentations in which the sex of the doctor or patient influenced the management, a study of the knowledge base for cardiac disease and the effect of gender, the effects of masculinity on patient presentations and on the experience of rural medicine, the experience of being a female rural doctor, stress management and acupuncture, and issues that attract women into rural medical practice. When students are not interested in rural practice, the tutorials reflect this by reviewing the general knowledge base and culture of medicine from a gender perspective. An evaluation of the unit is sought from each group of students. Content and structure of tutorials is modified in response to this feedback. Teaching staff at rural centres learnt to negotiate tutorial content with the students, and this was found to work well.

Teacher training. *Part of the tacit curriculum for the teaching is exposure of students to female rural doctors so they could see for themselves some of the ways it is possible to be a woman and a rural doctor. This required recruitment and training of practising rural doctors to the teaching team.* Initially only female doctors were identified to teach the course, but later male doctors were added, when the course changed from Women in Rural General Practice to Gender Issues for Rural Doctors. The author worked with each doctor individually to help them identify gendered knowledge and experience they could use as content for their tutorials. It was important not to require the tutors to develop theoretical expertise or wander too far from their grounded experience, as they had neither the time nor the inclination to do so. Each rural doctor identified experiences in which their gender played a part as a doctor, and patient presentations in which gender was a key ingredient in the presentation or management. Some doctors have a pre-existing interest and knowledge base, for example in gender and heart disease, or in gender and mental health and they were encouraged to build their tutorials around these interests and to combine gender analysis with the teaching of clinical skills. One teacher has an interest in acupuncture and stress management, and uses these skills as vehicles to teach about gender issues for rural doctors. Teaching this important curriculum unit is only possible because of the skill and generosity of the rural doctors who leave their surgeries and hospitals to teach the students on an honorary basis.

Faculty development. *The development of the curriculum was piloted before being introduced as core curriculum in 1998. This included the skilling of the teaching staff, and an opportunity to trial different approaches to content and presentation.* In most of the initial tutorials, the author was present to support the medical staff and to observe the interactions as a basis for further development. Teaching staff were provided with literature on the issues raised, and encouraged to test out a variety of case histories and observations about issues for women in rural practice, and later about gender issues for rural doctors.

One of the tutors took all three tutorials for the students in her hospital, and through this was able to explore the issues in greater depth and form a relationship with the students. At the other two hospitals, tutorial teams were developed and each member took one tutorial each three week rotation. It was important that the tutors briefed each other on what had been taught by them, and the level of interest in rural practice among the students. The author took one tutorial for each rotation at one of the hospitals, concentrating on developing a framework for the students to think about gender in medicine and its potential impact on their lives as doctors.

Develop teaching resources. *Teaching resources have been developed including case histories, personal experiences of female and male rural family doctors, select articles from published literature, and a theoretical framework considering gender issues in medicine.* Supplementary reading drawn from journal articles and the medical press provide take-away resources for the students to keep for a time when they are directly relevant to them.

What works. *The best tutorials are those that involve an exchange of experiences within the group, supported by the provision of an analytic framework within which to think about those experiences.* Discussions of case management led by an experienced family doctor were effective in involving the students in thinking about how sex and gender can influence the clinical interaction.

In the latter part of the year, students had already been on their general practice rotation. They were able to reflect on how male and female rural doctors managed their practice, the intersection of their personal and professional lives, and what that might mean for them as potential rural doctors.

There is some variability between the groups as to what works but in general, clinical case scenarios are well received, as is discussion of the tutor's personal experience. Giving students a range of options about what they would like to cover in the next tutorial is well received. An enthusiastic and positive approach is very important and modelling an enjoyment and passion for rural medical practice is helpful. Students comment that they do not have many chances to "see" people who work in rural medicine, especially women. Using examples and discussion points that are close to the students' own experience is helpful, and students particularly value the opportunity to discuss their expectations for the next year or two.

What does not work. *Aspects of the teaching that work less well include the introduction of theoretical consideration of gender issues in rural practice to groups comprised of all or predominantly urban, male students.* This proved especially difficult when the teachers were women. Students value an informal interactive approach but do not like tutorials where there is a lack of direction.

EVALUATION

At the end of each three week hospital rotation, students are asked to evaluate their teaching/learning experience, both as part of the general rural hospital curriculum, and as a specific evaluation of the gender curriculum. This feedback is incorporated into the development of materials and process for the next group of students. In 2001 this evaluation was replaced by a group interview. Students were briefly interviewed in same-sex groups, with a male interviewer present for the male students, and a female interviewer for the female students. They were asked "What have you learnt from the gender tutorials?" The discussion was tape-recorded and transcribed.

The most important response by the students was participation (Table 1). This was non-compulsory and non-examinable, and often close to their final exams. Most students took part, with women consistently more interested than men.

The written evaluation asked students to specify what worked and what did not work, for each of the three tutorials they were offered. Tables 2 and 3 provide a summary of the number and content of comments made by students in 1999 (from evaluation forms) and 2001 (from recorded discussions). Approximately 158 students were eligible to take part in the tutorials and the great majority did so.

TABLE 1. Participation by Students in Tutorials and Evaluation

	Participation Rate	Females	Males
Tutorial N = 86	83%	93%	65%
Evaluation N = 42	74%	84%	59%

The positive comments made by the students in Table 2 highlighted the value of having an opportunity to systematically consider questions that they were aware of for the most part, so they could develop the necessary vocabulary and test their ideas with their peers in the safety of a contained discussion. Many students appreciated the interactive nature of the teaching and the permission to speak about issues that are highly salient to some, yet they feel required to keep hidden. The objective of providing female students with female rural doctor role models has been achieved and was valued. Male and female students appreciated the extra insight into rural medical practice. Students were also asked "What did not work for you?" and there were some critical responses to the question "What have you learnt?" These are summarised in Table 3.

More than two-thirds of the comments by students were positive. For some women, it was very important to have a chance to explore the issues for women in rural medicine and medicine generally with the support of experienced staff. Other students, mostly male and including some of the women, found the topic upsetting and even became angry. The curriculum was developed around questions that had been raised by students, which gave it immediacy and saliency. It was, however, taught at a time when students were very exam focussed, and as a non-examinable component of the course, therefore students felt free to attend or not as their schedule permitted.

Students attending another hospital in the same year rated the tutorials at 4.2 on a scale of 1-5, with 5 being the most valued. One of the female students in 2001 contributed the following comment, providing some insight into the saliency and anxiety aroused by gender issues for students and doctors:

> *I think your tute allowed the rest of my group to acknowledge their agitation with the system. Their reactions over the last couple of days have been interesting to observe. The group attended a discussion on the accreditation of the Monash course and at the end of the session they decided to raise the issue of more female input, role models and alternative teaching methods, and put it into writing, an issue they would never have dreamed of raising in the past. Don't misinterpret me; I'm very proud of them but I'm worried that they aren't aware of the implications of their actions and I feel they could get burnt before they get much further. I ar-*

rived on the scene as they were handing in their suggestions and encour-
aged them to remove their names and contact details from the submission.
My reasons for this was that it was an accreditation body which is not a
group to be underestimated and I didn't know where and in whose hands
their names would end up.

Male students are often challenged by the teaching. Most of them do their best to learn from it, although a few react with hostility. The following comments were made during the group interview, and relate to the tutorial on issues for women in medicine in which, as a trial, the tutor separated the students into same-sex groups and asked them to identify the issues faced by female doctors. This tutorial was followed by one taken by a male doctor, concentrating on issues for men in rural medical practice:

Student A: When you say gender issues, I can feel that it's more relevant for women rather than for men because it's women that have more problems with gender discrimination and so especially the second tute we felt a bit out of it, it was a bit funny.

Student B: Yes. It was like 'you just go over there and sit there and talk,' and she kind of reacted with surprise every time we came up with something. You know, about the problems females have and that males actually know.

Student A: Yeah, because we came up with pretty much the points that the female group came up with, more or less. We were pretty proud of ourselves.

Student B: I think discussing it is different to learning as well but we did a lot of discussion. It was good discussion and it was a way of being able to see things and talk about them so we're more comfortable talking about them in the future so I suppose that's the biggest part . . . it was like just being able to put my opinions and know that they're kind of right and that I can express them and that sort of stuff.

In this discussion the men start by saying that gender was not a legitimate topic and they were left out, and end by saying they were proud they identified the same issues as the women, and that it helps them to be able to talk about it.

Changes were made to the teaching in response to the evaluations. The most important was to tailor the content of the tutorial to the sex balance of the tutorial group and the degree of interest in rural practice. It was found to be of little value to teach about issues for female rural doctors to a tutorial group comprised of males interested in urban-based super-specialities. It was necessary

TABLE 2. Evaluation of Gender Teaching for Final Year Medical Students During Their Rural Hospital Rotation: Responses to the Questions *What Worked? What Have You Learnt?*

Issues	Identified by the Students
Learning about professional identity N = 95 (30%)	Gender issues for doctors and patients (12%)
	Great session. As a Ballarat boy with a leaning towards general practice 'outside' Melbourne, this session was very relevant and inspiring. It was great to hear stories of personal experiences and get a feel of what to expect in the next few years 'on-the-job.' The sexual politics was, as per usual, a great topic to discuss.
	Got an appreciation of what differences men and women experience in practice from a personal and honest perspective which isn't readily discussed elsewhere.
	It (gender) is a hard topic to listen to but is very important to be aware of.
	Life as a rural doctor (11%)
	That was very interesting and worthwhile, that was good that discussion, was more about rural practice the pro's and con's and women's role in practice a little bit but it was more about rural.
	It was great to be able to discuss the issues that would face us in rural practice.
	Having a tutorial with a rural paediatrician who has a child of her own was a valuable experience.
	Being a female doctor (5%)
	I think also that it sort of inspired me in a way to think about making changes throughout my career despite the fact that I really am interested in a very male oriented field. I think that I would be able to make a difference if I was to become a surgeon I think that we could . . . start putting a female perspective on things and especially maybe also taking a role as a teacher and a leader so not just a private practitioner but to be also be involved in the training of other young female doctors.
	Good variety of different career paths which women took within the profession. It was informal so that was good.
	Learning about the lifestyle choices open to women in medicine.
	Becoming a doctor (2%)
	I enjoyed the laidback discussion of issues of becoming a doctor which are not discussed routinely.
	Discussion of intern life and further progress, relaxing atmosphere. The free discussion, dynamic session, sharing experience from the facilitator.
	Learning about male friendly specialties.
Content N = 66 (21%)	Interesting issues (12%)
	Interesting to have the issues raised and for us to be aware that these things happen. Liked an open forum of debate and discussion.
	Yeah it's made me more aware of it, I've found even in the last few days just being very conscious of what's happening around me and things like that.
	This was great and excellent. Chance to go outside hospital was good. And sensitive to our opinions.

Issues	Identified by the Students
	Good clinical teaching
	I liked it. It was very clinically orientated.
	Case studies were good discussion points. Discussion how to provide counselling to patients with psych. or sexual problems is rarely talked about elsewhere and using case examples was helpful.
	Very well done and much more informative than I had imagined.
	Complementary therapies
	Insight into complementary medicine was great.
	Excellent, a wonderful overview of alternative health and its role in today's medical services. Interesting and informative!
Learning environment N = 53 (17%)	Good discussion (14%)
	It was good to be able to discuss issues with someone who has done so much research in the area.
	Dr X was really great! Very open and I enjoyed hearing her experiences. It was great hearing about some of the things we may face and also the experiences and ideas of my colleagues.
	The openness of the session and willingness to discuss all issues.
	It was nice to have a chance to talk about it as well. I think it's something that goes unsaid. Because we are just expected to carry the flag and men are expected to bag the women, but it was nice actually being in the situation where you could talk about it.
	Safe environment (5%)
	Nice, comfortable environment. In fact they all created a very open and relaxing atmosphere.
	The freedom to say exactly what I thought without thinking I might be saying the wrong thing (i.e., the honesty).
	Being able freely to discuss very relevant issues in an honest way.
Total positive	There were 223 positive comments out of a total of 311 comments, or 72%.

to expand the content to include gender issues for men, and issues in medicine in general rather than just rural practice. This change was negotiated successfully with the funding body, although its primary purpose continues to be to facilitate interest among the female students in becoming rural family doctors. The most important evaluation by the students was that they attended the tutorials, which were non-compulsory and non-examinable, despite imminent final exams.

OUTCOME AT MONASH

Monash University has redeveloped its medical course and taught the new course for the first time in 2002, leading to modification of the gender teaching

TABLE 3. Evaluation of Gender Teaching for Final Year Medical Students During Their Rural Hospital Rotation: Responses to the Question *What Did Not Work?*

Issues	Identified by the Students
Content N = 55 (18%)	Not productive (5%) *The one man's issue was like putting up like you know a macho thing, there was really no benefit from it. I think we recognise that there are definite differences obviously in gender and there are issues that come up and gender collusions that occur.* *I don't think at our level final year, that you should have so much time spent on it, a lot of us and previous groups were saying it wasn't really beneficial for us.* *It did highlight the gender issue, however I didn't find it very productive.*
	Already know about it (4%) *Pointless divisive ear bashing raised some interesting issues but nothing I was not already aware of.* *Probably stuff you already knew but it does make us aware of it.* *I don't think you learn that much yourself but you might learn about other people's views. I think that's important.*
	Improve content (4%) *Talked too much about clinical trials and papers.* *I would have been more interested in finding out about her experience of being a rural doctor–the medical stuff we get a lot of!* *Good idea trying to explore whether or not doctors treat women or men differently, however I think that the examples didn't demonstrate this and therefore didn't lead into possible group discussion as to why.*
	Other suggestions (4%) *Was a good topic to bring up . . . we didn't really talk about solutions.* *None were especially relevant to me since I'm male and I'm not intending on marrying a doctor. Good for the girls, though.* *Having to refer to things as "male model" and "female model," we didn't really agree upon the premise of the lecture. Maybe the question should be posed "Do men and women practice differently?"*
Learning environment N = 33 (11%)	Alienated by presentation (5%) *It was quite offensive. I thought she'd taken it too far the other way. The way I approach gender issues is I think everyone should be treated equal, like sex comes into it but people are people.* *Interesting topic. I was disappointed at the way in which it was presented.* *I think she was insinuating that men have a better time in a hospital because they interact on a different social level with female nurses and other female professionals in the hospital, and we climb the hierarchical ladder that way rather than through professionalism and that really cheesed me off because that's not the way I do it. That may happen and it does happen to a certain extent, but that's not what I do.*

Issues	Identified by the Students
	Structure of teaching (4%)
	Difficult to create a dialogue/ask questions. Felt more like a didactic session.
	It was an interesting discussion, however at this time of year there are probably different issues of higher priority.
	One sided (2%)
	It was thought provoking to discuss these issues but quite one sided and extreme.
Total negative	28% of the total number of comments were negative or suggested improvements.

described above. The major outcome from learning in the development and implementation of gender teaching is the opportunity to mainstream gender sensitivity into the new curriculum. At the end of 2001, the Faculty Curriculum Committee established a Gender Working Party with a brief to contribute to the development of teaching material and a program of professional development to enhance staff awareness and skills in gender sensitive curriculum. Gender competency has been accepted as one of the core clinical skills students must acquire and they will receive teaching about gender and health throughout the course. Gender will continue to feature as part of the rural curriculum, both through a rural gender case that was the basis of learning for the students for two weeks in Semester 3, and a one day seminar. This is only possible because there now exists a group of academic and honorary staff skilled in gender teaching.

Other Universities

Teaching about gender in medical curriculum is only sustainable if there is a national and international constituency supporting the concept. Much work has been devoted to developing this constituency. Staff have been identified at other universities who are passionate and knowledgeable about issues for women as rural doctors or gender issues in medicine, and five additional universities now employ part-time staff to introduce this teaching into their rural curriculum.

CREATING LEGITIMACY OF TEACHING ABOUT GENDER ISSUES IN MEDICINE

The Monash team has consistently presented the issues to national and international medical meetings, and identified and trained leading academic and medical women in the knowledge base and vocabulary required to assert the legitimacy of the teaching. International work has included workshops held under the auspices of the World Organisation of Family Doctors (WONCA), resulting in various policy changes and increased attention to gender (Chater 2000; Wainer 2000). In addition, the meeting of the Medical Women's International Association in Sydney in 2001 included a session on Women in Medicine, and international symposium on Teaching Gendered Medicine (Wainer & Nobelius 2002). Work continues in Australia with workshops and seminars held at a national level (Wainer 1999). The Australian College of Rural and Remote Medicine included in its foundation Prospectus policy on Women in Rural Practice (ACRRM 1997) and the chair of the Women in Rural Practice Committee is a member of the Board.

A survey of female rural doctors in the state of Victoria was conducted by Monash University School of Rural Health (Wainer 2001), following a similar survey in the state of New South Wales (McEwin 2001), and another in Queensland (White & Fergusson 2001). These are building the evidence base on which to further develop curriculum and policy. Residential workshops have also been held to a variety of audiences (Wainer et al. 1999; Wainer 2000; Wainer, Greacen & Ginnane 2001) and workshops presented at state and regional rural doctor conferences. This has all been essential work to develop the issues, test them for validity and saliency, refine the framework and vocabulary, and identify networks of doctors skilled and interested to develop the theory and implement it in practice.

CONCLUSION

This foundation work completed to introduce teaching about gender issues for doctors has created the discipline of Gendered Medicine. It draws on the great body of work by women's health theorists and researchers around the world, and the less robust but developing work of the men's health movement. An essential condition of this work is that it met an identified learning need of the medical students, a workforce planning need of the funders, and a political imperative identified by the Commonwealth Government. As discussed, the issue was also relevant for students, including the need of female students to meet and talk with female doctors. The initiative required authorisation and support from senior medical academic men, and courageous and persistent work from senior medical academic women. With that authorisation and support, backed up by funding, it is both possible and necessary to systematically teach medical students about the gender issues embedded in the knowledge base, research programes, professional structures, training programes and careers of doctors.

REFERENCES

ACRRM (1997). *Prospectus Australian College of Rural and Remote Medicine*, Kelvin Grove, Queensland.

Australian Medical Workforce Advisory Committee & Australian Institute of Health and Welfare (1996). *Female Participation in The Australian Medical Workforce*, Sydney, AAMWAC Report 1996.7.

Australian Medical Workforce Advisory Committee (AMWAC) (1998). *Influences on Participation in the Australian Medical Workforce*, Sydney: AMWAC. Report 1998.4.

Britt H, Bhasale A, Miles D, Meza A, Sayer G, Angelis M (1996). *The Sex of the General Practitioner: A Comparison of Characteristics, Patients and Medical Conditions Managed*. Medical Care, 34(5), 403-15.

Britt H (1999). *Bettering the Evaluation and Care of Health: General Practice Activity in Australia (1998-99)*, Australian Institute of Health and Welfare, Canberra.

Brown W, Young A, Byles J (1997). *Women's Health Australia: A Health Profile of Mid-Life Rural Women* in the Proceedings of the National Rural Public Health Forum, Deakin West, ACT, National Rural Health Alliance.

Bundrock V (1996). *Gippsland Women's Health: Report of a Survey*. Churchill, Victoria, Australia, Monash University.

Carson D, Stringer K (1998). *Generation and Gender Issues: The Emerging Culture Within the Rural and Remote Medical Workforce* proceedings of the 4th Biennial Australian Rural and Remote Health Scientific Conference, Cunningham Centre, Toowoomba.

Chater B (ed) (2000). *World Organisation of Family Doctors Policy on Rural Practice and Rural Health*, Monash University School of Rural Health, Traralgon, Victoria.

De Angelis, CD (2000). *Women in Academic Medicine: New Insights, Same Sad News*, The New England Journal of Medicine, 342(6), February 10.

Hanemaaijer I (1995). National Rural Undergraduate Medical Conference Report on Behalf of Rural Undergraduate Steering Committee, Department of Health and Aged Care, Commonwealth of Australia, Canberra.

Hanemaaijer I (1995). *Undergraduate Rural Curriculum Conference August 1994 Report*, Commonwealth Department of Human Services and Health, Canberra.

Hojat M, Gonnella J, Xu G (1995). *Gender Comparisons of Young Physicians' Perceptions of Their Medical Education, Professional Life, and Practice: A Follow-Up Study of Jefferson Medical College Graduates*, Academic Medicine, 70(4), April.

Levitt L, McEwin K (2001). *Wanted: New Rural Workforce Strategies for Female Doctors: Findings from a Survey of Women in Rural Medicine*, NSW Rural Doctors Network, Mascot, Australia.

Makan B (1998). Distribution of Health Personnel, *South African Health Review*, Health Services Trust, *www.hst.org.za/sahr/98/chap7.htm*

McEwin K (2001). *Wanted: New Rural Workforce Strategies for Female Doctors–Findings from a Survey of Women in Rural Medicine* NSW Rural Doctors Network, Mascot, NSW.

Moodley K, Barnes JM, de Villiers PJT (1999). *Constraints Facing the Female Medical Practitioner in Private Family Practice in the Western Cape*, South African Medical Journal, 89(2), February, 165-169.

Redman S, Saltman D, Straton J, Young B, Paul C (1994). *Determinants of Career Choice Among Women and Men Medical Students and Interns*, Medical Education, 28(5).

Rogers S (1995). *Women in the Medical Workforce*, Commonwealth Department of Human Services and Health.

Rourke LL, Rourke J, Brown JB (1996). *Women Family Physicians in Rural Medicine: Can the Grass be Greener in the Country?* Canadian Family Physician, 42, 1063-1067, 1077-1082.

Rourke J, Strasser R (1996). *Education for Rural Practice in Canada and Australia* Academic Medicine, 71(5), May, 464-469.

Schei B (1996). *Curriculum Development for Postgraduate Training in Psychosocial Obstetrics and Gynaecology*, Paper presented to the Second International Conference on Teaching to Promote Women's Health, Toronto.

Strasser R, Kamien M, Hays R, Carson D (1997). *National Rural General Practice Study*, Monash University Centre for Rural Health, Traralgon.

Strasser RP (1992). *Rural General Practice in Victoria: The Report from A Study of the Attitudes of Victorian General Practitioners to Country Practice and Training*, Department of Community Medicine, Monash University, Melbourne.

Thompson D. (1997). *Can We Cope with Life in a Rural Town ? Issues of Concern to Rural Training Stream Registrars*, Paper presented to the 2nd World Rural Health Congress, Durbin.

Tolhurst H, Bell P, Baker L, Talbot J, Cleasby L (1997). *Educational and Support Needs of Female Rural General Practitioners*, School of Nursing and Health Administration, Charles Sturt University, Bathurst.

Turner J, Tippett V, Raphael B. (1994). *Women in Medicine–Socialization, Stereotypes and Self-Perceptions*, Australian and New Zealand Journal of Psychiatry, 28, 129-135

Wainer J (1998). *Rural Women's Health*, Australian Journal of Primary Health–Interchange, 4(3).

Wainer J (1999). *Teaching Gender Seminar*, Monash University School of Rural Health, Traralgon, Victoria.

Wainer J, Bryant L, Carson D, Strasser R, Stringer K (1999). *A Life, Not a Wife*, Proceedings of the 5th National Rural Health Conference, Adelaide.

Wainer J, Carson D, Strasser R (2000). *Women and Rural Medical Practice*, South African Family Practice Journal, 22(6), 19-23.

Wainer J (2000) *Global Issues in Rural Women's Health*, Proceedings of The WONCA 3rd World Conference on Rural Health, Acadamy of Family Physicians of Malaysia, Kuala Lumpur, pp. 59-65.

Wainer J (2000). *'New Voices in Rural Medical Practice,'* in *5th Biennial Australian Rural Remote Health Scientific Conference–Infront Outback*, Conference Proceedings, Abstract, Toowoomba, QLD.

Wainer J (2001). *Female Rural Doctors in Victoria: It's Where We Live*, Rural Workforce Agency, Melbourne, Victoria, May 2001, 71.

Wainer J, Greacen J, Ginnane J (2001). *'Victorian Rural Women Practitioner Survey,'* in *6th National Rural Health Conference, Incorporating Infront Outback*–'Good Health ~ Good Country from Conception to Completion, 4-7 March 2001, National Convention Centre Canberra.' National Rural Health Alliance, Canberra. Non-Refereed Published Paper (CD Rom).

White C, Fergusson S (2001). *Female Medical Practitioners in Rural and Remote Queensland: An analysis of Findings, Issues and Trends*, Queensland Rural Medical Support Agency, Kelvin Grove, Queensland.

Outing Lesbian Health
in Medical Education

Ruth McNair, MBBS, DRACOG, DA(UK), FRACGP, FACRRM

SUMMARY. Lesbian health is emerging as a distinct discipline in practice and research. Evidence is increasingly available that lesbians are a unique and underserved population in the health care system. They display reduced health seeking behaviors and have specific risk factors which potentially affect their health and well being. They also have specific health issues in fields as diverse as fertility, sexual health and mental health, which require specific knowledge from health care practitioners. Above all, lesbian health care consumers repeatedly decry the lack of sensitivity and knowledge that they experience in their interactions with providers, and call for improved training. However, medical education generally ignores lesbian health at all levels. In this paper, the inclusion of lesbian health in medical education programs is reviewed, and recent political initiatives involving gay and lesbian health in Australia are dis-

Ruth McNair is Senior Lecturer and Director of Undergraduate Education, Department of General Practice, University of Melbourne. She was awarded The University of Melbourne Cultural Diversity Award (Academic Staff) in 2000. Dr. McNair is currently conducting research on lesbian parenting. She practices part-time in an inner-urban general practice, with a focus on women's health, and lesbian health. Dr. McNair is a member of the Victorian Ministerial Advisory Committee on Gay and Lesbian Health, and the Victorian Attorney General's Committee on Gay, Lesbian and Transgender Issues, and is Convener of the Australian Lesbian Medical Association.

Address correspondence to: Ruth McNair, University of Melbourne, 200 Berkeley Street, Carlton, Victoria 3053, Australia (E-mail: r.mcnair@unimelb.edu.au).

[Haworth co-indexing entry note]: "Outing Lesbian Health in Medical Education." McNair, Ruth. Co-published simultaneously in *Women & Health* (The Haworth Medical Press, an imprint of The Haworth Press, Inc.) Vol. 37, No. 4, 2003, pp. 89-103; and: *Teaching Gender, Teaching Women's Health: Case Studies in Medical and Health Science Education* (ed: Lenore Manderson) The Haworth Medical Press, an imprint of The Haworth Press, Inc., 2003, pp. 89-103. Single or multiple copies of this article are available for a fee from The Haworth Document Delivery Service [1-800-HAWORTH, 9:00 a.m. - 5:00 p.m. (EST). E-mail address: docdelivery@haworthpress.com].

cussed. The paper concludes with suggestions to integrate lesbian health in medical training. *[Article copies available for a fee from The Haworth Document Delivery Service: 1-800-HAWORTH. E-mail address: <docdelivery@ haworthpress.com> Website: <http://www.HaworthPress.com> © 2003 by The Haworth Press, Inc. All rights reserved.]*

KEYWORDS. Lesbian health, medical education, barriers to health care, marginalization within medicine

INTRODUCTION

   Lesbian health is achieving status as a legitimate discipline of health care practice and research. The Council of Scientific Affairs of the American Medical Association (1996) updated its policy regarding gay men and lesbians in 1994. The Council suggested that optimal patient care is compromised when doctors fail to recognize that a patient is lesbian or gay, called for nonjudgemental recognition of sexual orientation and behavior, and recommends that the subject of homosexuality be included in the education of all students in medical school. The growth of the lesbian health movement in the USA is also evidenced by the release of a comprehensive discussion document on lesbian health by the Institute of Medicine (Solarz, 2000). One of its eight recommendations was that health professional associations and academic institutions "should develop and support mechanisms for broadly disseminating information and knowledge about lesbian health to health care providers, researchers and the public" (ibid.: 14).

   Culturally aware health care is increasingly being recognized as important at a political level. In September 2000 the Parliamentary Assembly of the Council of Europe, representing 41 European countries, voted overwhelmingly for a series of recommendations supporting gay and lesbian rights. These included a recommendation that positive measures be taken to combat homophobic attitudes, especially in the medical profession, schools, armed forces and police, by means of training. At a national policy level in the USA, lesbians and gay men are included in target groups for reducing health inequalities in the government's 10-year plan for public health (USDHHS, 2000). Public health research is also embracing the area, with a special issue of the *American Journal of Public Health* on lesbian, gay, bisexual and transgender health in June 2001. This is the first time that this theme has been featured, and met with large numbers of submissions (Northridge, 2001).

   In Australia, there is some recognition of the need for policy development with respect to gay and lesbian health, with the establishment of advisory committees in the states of Victoria and Tasmania in 2000. Victoria is currently reviewing its Women's Health and Wellbeing policy and has identified lesbians as one of 5 target groups for special consideration. The South Australian Department of Human Services (2000) released a Women's Health and Wellbeing consultation paper in December 2000, and while lesbians are not specifically targeted, one of the eight 'critical issues' listed is sexuality. This paper includes a brief discussion of barriers to quality care affecting lesbian and bisexual women including diversity, discrimination, homophobia, coming out, heterosexism, and health care provider lack of information and discomfort.

The Australian Medical Association has produced a position statement on sexuality and gender diversity which includes the need for improved education by health care providers in this area. In this paper, the evidence for the need to recognise lesbian health as a specific discipline within medical education and research is presented.

KNOWLEDGE OF LESBIAN HEALTH

Health care professionals require specific teaching related to lesbian health issues and inequalities (Moran, 1996; Lehmann, Lehmann and Kelly, 1998). Lesbian patients are very aware that their doctors lack knowledge in this area, and public submissions received by the Victorian Ministerial Advisory Committee on Gay and Lesbian Health in 2000 revealed education of health care providers to be the most commonly raised issue of concern (McNair, Anderson and Mitchell, 2001). Harrison states that "the vast majority of physicians surveyed feel that they have not received adequate education and training in human sexuality in medical school and nothing in homosexuality"(1996:18), and claims that medical students prefer that gay and lesbian issues be integrated throughout the entire medical school curriculum. Another study of psychiatrists' and general practitioners' attitudes to gay men showed that these doctors believed that their education on sexuality had been "woefully inadequate" (King, 1994: 854).

Areas of knowledge requiring lesbian cultural sensitivity and knowledge include issues relating to mental health, reproductive health, gynaecological care, sexual health, and drug and alcohol use. Older lesbians' needs are neglected by social and health services, as the services continue to assume that clients are heterosexual. Harrison (1999) suggests that the recognition of sexuality as a cultural identity in aged care is the way forward, much as aboriginality is now becoming recognised within the aged care sector. She discusses the need for the lesbian community to control the changes required, and the need for education within the health sector. At any age, isolation and a lack of connectedness to a community are major risk factors for mental health problems such as depression and anxiety. An Australian Drug Foundation study into gay and lesbian drug and alcohol use revealed an alarming trend amongst lesbians towards maintaining higher levels of drug, alcohol and tobacco intake as they got older (Murnane et al., 2000). Certain cancers such as breast and ovarian cancer may be more prevalent among older lesbians due to a predominance of risk factors such as non-childbearing, smoking, and inadequate screening (Rankow, 1995), although data for Australian lesbians regarding their prevalence of risk factors for such conditions are not currently available. There is generally a lack of Australian population-based data comparing the health issues of lesbians with the general population. Providers' knowledge must therefore be based on international information until Australian data becomes available.

BARRIERS TO QUALITY HEALTH CARE FOR LESBIANS

Negative attitudes amongst health care providers towards lesbians impact on the quality of health care for this group. Lesbians are reported to display reduced health-seeking behavior including avoidance of routine health care (Harrison, 1996), delay in seeking health care (Trippet and Bain, 1992; Saphira and Glover, 2000), less frequent screening such as Pap testing (Smith, Johnson and Guenther, 1985; Carroll, 1999), and avoidance of disclosure of sexual orientation (Mathieson, 1998), due to negative medical attitudes and lack of specific knowledge regarding lesbian health. Lesbian consumer research repeatedly reveals dissatisfaction with medical care and perceptions of discriminatory attitudes and behavior of health care providers including doctors (Bradford, 1994; Trippet and Bain, 1992; Moran, 1996; White and Dull, 1997; Saphira and Glover, 2000). These consumer surveys show that between 31% and 89% of health care professionals displayed negative reactions to the revelation that their patients were gay or lesbian. The wide range reflects the variety of consumers surveyed, their expectations, and previous experiences of negative attitudes. Previous negative experiences tend to sensitize the patient to even subtle displays of homophobia or heterosexist assumptions in the practitioner, which include embarrassment, inappropriate responses, rejection of patients, hostility, and excessive curiosity, pity or condescension (Harrison, 1996:12). A Victorian survey of over 900 lesbian, gay, bisexual and transgender people reveals that 23% had experienced discrimination when accessing medical care (VGLRL, 2000).

Discriminatory attitudes of medical professionals towards lesbian patients have also been demonstrated through surveys of doctors. One survey revealed that 23% of doctors were severely homophobic, 60% homophobic overall and 40% uncomfortable treating lesbians and gay men (Mathews et al., 1986). A 1994 survey of 711 members of the USA-based Gay and Lesbian Medical Association showed that 52% of respondents had observed colleagues providing reduced care or denying care to patients because of their sexual orientation, and 88% reported hearing colleagues make disparaging remarks about lesbian, gay and bisexual patients (Schatz and O'Hanlan, 1994). A similar survey of 55 members of the Australian Lesbian Medical Association (response rate 82%) carried out by the author in 2001 replicated the American data, with 36% having observed colleagues denying care and 89% having heard disparaging remarks by colleagues about lesbian and gay patients.

Medical attitudes need not be overtly negative to create barriers. Assumptions of heterosexuality are frequently reported by lesbian consumers (Mathieson, 1998), as are health care workers' perceptions that they have few, if any, lesbian patients (Horsley and Tremellen, 1996; Berkman and Zinberg, 1997; McNair, 2000). Most practitioners are reluctant to facilitate disclosure of lesbian sexuality by their patients, preferring to leave the responsibility for disclosure with the patient. At The Royal Women's Hospital, Melbourne, 52 of 64 members of the nursing and medical staff reported that they would never ask a woman if she were lesbian (Brown, 2000). Stevens (1995) argues that the health care system is heterosexist in both its structure and the attitudes of individual providers, which competes with the provider's otherwise supportive interactions with lesbians. This heterosexism, combined with the reluctance of many lesbians to disclose, creates an invisibility which prevents doctors from understanding the full contextual perspective for these patients.

MEDICAL ATTITUDES LEADING TO MARGINALIZATION OF LESBIAN MEDICAL STUDENTS AND DOCTORS

Lesbian doctors and medical students as well as patients face discrimination and homophobia adversely affecting their well being. Fifty-four percent of lesbian doctors and medical students in the USA have experienced discrimination within the medical profession as a result of their sexual orientation (Schatz and O'Hanlan, 1994), as have 47% of Australian Lesbian Medical Association members. This is predominantly due to negative attitudes and behavior of colleagues. A 1986 survey of doctors' attitudes showed that 30% doctors interviewed were opposed to admitting gays and lesbians to medical schools and 40% would not refer clients to gay or lesbian colleagues (Matthews et al., 1986). A more recent study in New Mexico shows a positive shift in attitudes, with only 4.3% saying they would refuse gay and lesbian applicants admission to medical school (Ramos et al., 1998). However, research carried out in 1993 in the United States involving 4,501 female doctors showed that 41% of lesbian/bisexual doctors (n = 156) experienced harassment related to their sexual orientation, compared to 10% of heterosexual doctors (n = 4,177) (Brogan et al., 1999).

Lesbian and gay medical students and doctors experience invisibility, marginalization and discrimination for the same reasons as lesbian and gay patients (Tinmouth and Hamwi, 1994; Bambas, 1996). They face assumptions of heterosexuality by their colleagues, disparaging remarks and harassment, and consequently develop fears of negative impact on career progression if their sexual orientation is revealed (Brogan et al., 1999; Saunders, Oxley and Harvey, 2000). Lesbian and gay medical students and residents attempt to match their selection of residency placement to one in which they will feel welcomed and respected, yet still fear discrimination if they come out (Oriel et al., 1996). Their sexual orientation affects their choice of career path and a great deal of energy is expended "trying to find a balance between self-protection and self-disclosure" in making that choice (Risdon et al., 2000: 334). Most lesbian and gay doctors report that they do not disclose their sexual orientation within their profession due to fear of ostracism (Rose, 1994; Saunders et al., 2000). This creates a sense of discomfort in failing to be completely honest, yet is weighed up against the need to maintain safety (Risdon et al., 2000).

Medical students are especially vulnerable to the affects of negative attitudes, as they are often just coming to terms with their sexuality and fear the consequences of disclosure within their course (Tinmouth and Hamwi, 1994). They also want a more affirming study experience, including the incorporation of gay and lesbian issues into all coursework (Townsend et al., 1991). They do not see their own lives represented in any of the course material. Marginalization of lesbian and gay doctors, medical students and faculty staff is inextricably related to the exclusion of lesbian and gay health in medical education and a resultant failure of medical school curricula to challenge any negative attitudes that may exist.

METHODS FOR IMPROVING THE WELL-BEING OF SEXUALITY MINORITIES WITHIN MEDICINE

Inclusion of lesbian and gay health into medical curricula will assist in reducing the marginalization of lesbian and gay medical students. This education should include specific areas of knowledge, skills for sensitive communication and positive attitudes towards lesbian and gay patients and colleagues (Robinson and Cohen, 1996; Johnson and Henderson 2000). Beyond the educational framework, universities can also protect their students by developing guidelines on anti-discrimination that include sexual orientation and advocating for legislative reform in this regard (Schatz and O'Hanlan, 1994). Only 10% of UK medical schools have specific policies protecting medical students against discrimination (Bewley and Bolton, 1999). The British Gay and Lesbian Association of Doctors and Dentists (GLADD) workshop on challenging workplace bullying and homophobia in the NHS addressed the need for national guidelines addressing homophobia (Saunders, 2001).

A further method to improve the well-being of lesbian and gay students and doctors is to create specific support systems (Bambas, 1996). A national survey of support services for gay students in United States medical schools in 1990 showed that approximately half the medical schools had a specific support group (Townsend et al., 1991). A repeat survey in 1994 showed that 70% had a support group and nine schools had an official gay and lesbian liaison officer, compared with four in 1990 (Townsend et al., 1996). At the postgraduate level, lesbian and gay doctors' associations can create links and much needed support (Saunders et al., 2000). Associations exist in several countries including USA (Simpson, 1997), UK, France, Germany, Sweden, Norway, Switzerland, and Canada (GLMA, 2000). The Australian Lesbian Medical Association was formed in 1999. This is the first such national association in Australia, providing support and connection for over 120 lesbian doctors and medical students and advocacy for lesbian health issues. These groups enable mentoring within the profession for sexuality minorities, by providing support to disclose sexual orientation within the workplace. By disclosing their sexuality these doctors can then become role models for others (Burke and White, 2001).

INTERNATIONAL EDUCATION REGARDING LESBIAN HEALTH– ATTITUDES

Medical education traditionally focuses on the acquisition of knowledge and skills for medical practice. Education designed to influence student attitudes is now gaining ground as a legitimate domain, with an understanding that attitudes can be shaped through education. The General Medical Council (GMC) in the United Kingdom established goals of knowledge, skills and attitudes for undergraduate medical education in 1993: "The student should acquire and demonstrate attitudes necessary for the achievement of high standards of medical practice, both in the provision of care to individuals and populations and to his (sic) own personal development" (cited in Johnson and Henderson, 2000:589). The objectives for achievement of this goal include recognition and respect for difference. Johnson and Henderson (ibid) suggest that the application of these objectives with regard to homosexuality is especially challenging, in part due to the interweaving of direct personal relevance for students.

There is some evidence that negative attitudes towards homosexuality can be altered through educational interventions. Bauman and Hale (1985) established an elective course for first year medical students to promote positive attitudes towards gay and lesbian patients. This involved discussion of specific medical issues through small group interactions with gay and lesbian people.

A fifteen-scale attitude questionnaire was administered before and after the elective. The study group became significantly more accepting of homosexual lifestyles than the control group. A more recent study involved first year medical students at Louisiana State University (Wallick et al., 1995). On entry to the course, the students completed a 25-item questionnaire regarding their attitudes to homosexuals, then repeated the survey following a panel presentation by gay and lesbian people, at the end of first year, then during third year. They found that the students' interactions with the panel reduced stereotypical attitudes, although over time without any further education the attitudes rebounded slightly. Small group discussion created awareness amongst students that negative attitudes could adversely affect their clinical judgment.

An elective course in attitudes toward homosexuality at the University of Cambridge, UK demonstrates a teaching method for encouraging attitudinal change (Johnson and Henderson, 2000). Small groups of third year students with a facilitator explored common words used to describe lesbian and gay people and then explored the discrimination and stereotyping inherent within these words. Students were then asked to imagine how they would feel facing these attitudes as a lesbian or gay man and what behaviour they would display in response, raising issues such as avoidance, internalized homophobia and militancy, and the potential for fluidity of emotions and behaviors over time. Finally, students were asked how this understanding would apply to their future medical practice. Student comments from the evaluations are described and demonstrate insights into prejudicial attitudes and desires to incorporate new understandings into their personal life.

MEDICAL EDUCATION REGARDING LESBIAN HEALTH ISSUES– KNOWLEDGE AND SKILLS

National reviews of undergraduate medical course gay and lesbian content have been conducted in the USA (Wallick, 1992; Tesar and Rovi, 1998) and Britain (Bewley and Bolton, 1999) and Canada (Robb, 1996b). All reveal limited time-allocation and poorly integrated teaching regarding lesbian and gay health issues, with a tendency to teach about sexual orientation within an illness framework. None address lesbian health specifically. A survey of all 126 US medical schools via psychiatry departments had a 65% response rate (Wallick, 1992), of which 8 of 82 responding schools reported no teaching in lesbian and gay health, and the average time of teaching for the rest was three and a half hours for the whole course. Most taught through lecture(s) on sexuality, 40% via small group meetings with gay and lesbian people or panels, and almost a third used case vignettes. The conclusions were that the topic was marginalised and that homosexuality should be integrated throughout the curriculum.

Similarly, in a study of all 116 USA medical schools with a family medicine department (82% response rate), 50% reported no teaching on gay and lesbian issues, and the average time devoted to such issues over the four-year course was 2.5 hours (Tesar and Rovi, 1998). The main teaching method was lectures in medical ethics and in sexuality. The authors recommend integration of lesbian and gay health issues within curriculum, although specific issues may be lost if certain topics are not taught separately.

In Canada, several barriers to the inclusion of gay and lesbian issues exist in undergraduate medical courses, including assumptions that problem-based learning (PBL) cases should be heterosexual unless HIV is the subject (Robb, 1996b). Lesbian health in particular is found to be absent within curricula. Gay men's health beyond HIV has some exposure, a contrast which Robb credits to the more highly politicized nature of gay men's health. The invisibility of lesbian health is highlighted by its treatment in the referencing system Index Medicus, in which 'lesbian' is listed as 'see homosexuality' and 'homosexuality' is related to HIV/AIDS. Robb also observes that local champions tend to drive curriculum inclusion rather than an overriding framework, although this approach can create valuable mentoring and role modelling by gay and lesbian academics, creating attitudinal change. In response, an editorial (Robinson and Cohen, 1996) proposes a framework for all Canadian medical schools to include four components integrating knowledge, attitudes and skills:

1. didactic teaching of knowledge;
2. small groups to explore attitudes, share concerns, allow gay and lesbian students to feel safe;
3. use of simulated patients to develop skills in sensitive history taking; and
4. supervised interviews with real gay and lesbian patients.

Finally, a survey of medical and dental schools in the UK showed that only 40% taught anything relating to gay and lesbian issues (Bewley and Bolton, 1999). These were taught in genitourinary, psychiatry, communication skills and sexuality subjects.

LESBIAN HEALTH INCLUSION
IN MEDICAL EDUCATION IN AUSTRALIA

The Australian Medical Council (AMC) is the national standards body for primary medical training, involved in curriculum review and accreditation of each Australian medical school. Following the British lead, the AMC (2001) has established three goals relating to knowledge and understanding, skills, and attitudes as they affect professional behavior. The AMC recognizes the importance of formal teaching in professional attitudes and has encouraged specific streams for teaching and assessing attitudes in new courses at Flinders University, the University of Melbourne and the University of Queensland. Several AMC objectives incorporate issues relevant to lesbian health and the lesbian patient, although none specifically refer to sexual orientation. Under the knowledge and understanding goal, one objective regards knowledge of factors affecting *human relationships*, the psychological well being of patients and their families, and the *interactions between humans and their social* and physical environment (italics added). A second objective relates to knowledge of methods of meeting the health care *needs of disadvantaged groups* within the community. A skills objective includes the ability to communicate clearly, *considerately and sensitively* with patients, relatives, doctors, nurses, other health professionals and the general public. Finally, two of the attitudes objectives are respect for every human being, with an *appreciation of the diversity* of human background and cultural values; and recognition that the *health interests of the patients* and the community are paramount.

Data have not been collected systematically on the extent to which lesbian and gay issues are included within Australian medical curricula, but anecdotal evidence suggests very little teaching in this area. A survey of 64 medical and nursing staff at the Royal Women's Hospital, Melbourne showed that only 38% rated themselves as well informed regarding lesbian health, with 63% expressing a willingness to learn more (Brown, 2000). Gay men's issues are predominantly presented in the context of HIV/AIDS; lesbian health simply has not rated a mention. As reported in international literature, lesbian students and doctors are highly aware of the lack of representation of issues pertaining to their own cultural context and actively seek any reference to lesbian issues within their courses. Half of the members of the Australian Lesbian Medical Association had not received any education regarding lesbian issues, and those who had received such teaching recalled an average of 2.4 hours relating to lesbian health at undergraduate level. Only 11% recalled teaching at the postgraduate level and 3.5% in the workplace, both for an average of 2 hours (McNair unpublished survey, 2001).

New medical curricula are spreading across Australian universities using a PBL format, early clinical exposure and a systems-based approach replacing discipline-specific teaching. This should create an opportunity to include lesbian issues, at the very least by generating cases using lesbians, or lesbian relatives and friends. A gender review of cases used in PBL at The University of Newcastle, however, reveals not only that the gender of cases is not representative of the community in general, but that very few cases are lesbian (Helen Tolhurst, personal communication). An audit by the author of the first two years of cases used in PBL at the University of Melbourne regarding gender, rurality, ethnicity and sexuality, reveals no gay or lesbian cases at all. This clearly points to a lack of a systematic approach with regard to representation of minority issues.

The University of Adelaide is developing a new medical curriculum using largely student-directed learning through contextual PBL, and has developed one such systematic approach (Laraine Ruthborn, personal communication). Twenty concept mapping groups were convened, one of which is for gay and lesbian content, to identify what concepts should be included in the curriculum (to define the content) and how and when these concepts should be covered (to ensure vertical and horizontal integration). As the committee on gay and lesbian content worked through the task, it became obvious that staff behaviour and attitudes would be crucial in determining the success of student learning in this area. Role modelling by staff members is powerful in establishing and/or changing student attitudes and beliefs, and it is likely that staff members would represent the wide range of attitudes towards homosexuality found in society itself. The need for staff development was established, so that cases are presented and facilitated appropriately, ensuring that heterosexist or homophobic remarks by staff or students are challenged appropriately. Strategies to encourage staff to attend heterosexism/homophobia workshops are being developed.

RECOMMENDATIONS FOR AUSTRALIAN MEDICAL SCHOOLS

Each medical school should make a commitment to include sexuality minority issues as a priority within medical education, just as governments around the country are starting to endorse policy development in this area. This should sit within a social model of health, where the issues are raised within the broader biopsychosocial context. This will enable student understanding of the lesbian patient's perspective, where dealing with homophobic attitudes, heterosexism, isolation and family rejection are universal experiences and create many of the specific health issues and risk factors for this population. It will broaden the understanding of differing health seeking behaviors amongst lesbians, which have been exacerbated by actual or expected negative experiences within the medical system.

Lesbian issues should be integrated throughout curricula systematically, ideally facilitated by a curriculum overview committee designated to track insertion of sexuality minority issues throughout each of the domains of the course. Ensuring that there is a representative sample of lesbians within PBL cases, either as the case itself or as a relative or carer, is a simple first step. This would allow lesbian issues to be raised in the context of bio-scientific subject material, a subject often seen by students and faculty as the most important. Care must be taken when presenting lesbian patients that their issues are not stereotyped or pathologised. For example, the higher incidence of attempted suicide amongst young lesbians should be addressed, however the underlying trigger should be emphasised as the negative societal or family attitudes, rather than lesbianism per se. In the same way, lesbian drug and alcohol misuse can be raised as an important risk behavior associated with a marginalized group.

In the domain of professional attitudes and development, exploring attitudes towards lesbians in society can be juxtaposed against the impact of those attitudes on lesbians and the literature around negative experiences within the medical system. This will challenge students to assess their own attitudes and modifications that may be required. In the health and society domain, gender issues and women's health are often included. These can be expanded to include sexual orientation, sexual behaviour and sexual identity as three interweaving experiences for patients. Issues of confidentiality regarding sexual orientation in dealing with adolescents and adults who are just coming out should also be addressed. Finally, in the clinical skills domain, awareness raising regarding common assumptions of heterosexuality is important with subsequent skills building regarding the use of inclusive language and a non-judgemental approach.

CONCLUSION

There is a need to educate medical students and doctors about lesbian health to remove well-documented barriers to quality health care for lesbians. Until then, lesbian patients will continue to encounter doctors with little specific knowledge, inadequate communication skills and discriminatory attitudes. An imperative for curricular inclusion of lesbian health is also generated by the needs of lesbians within the medical profession, for whom curricula silence perpetuates marginalization.

In Australia, we face several barriers to the introduction of lesbian health into curricula. Key barriers exist at the curriculum development level including the lack of a systematic approach or framework by which to teach the subject, and consequent reliance on local champions. The teaching of attitudes is in its infancy in medical education, despite good evidence that this is effective. Issues such as homophobia and heterosexism remain difficult to tackle. Finally, there is a lack of recognition that lesbian health is a distinct discipline with its own health inequalities and risk factors, evidenced by the lack of local research and its absence in Australian medical literature. There is also a need for medical schools, specialist colleges and hospitals to support lesbian and gay staff and students by having anti-discrimination policies and processes in place. Staff development programs including anti-homophobia and anti-heterosexism training should be instituted, as should visible and accessible support systems for lesbian and gay staff and students.

Political changes are occurring, including recognition of the need for lesbian and gay health care policy by some Australian state governments. Australian doctors are not prepared for this ground swell and must look to international developments. Lesbian health issues are slowly permeating into medical curricula internationally and in Australia there is an excellent opportunity as new undergraduate courses are being developed. Only then will we provide a safe environment for lesbian students and quality health care for lesbian patients.

REFERENCES

Australian Medical Council. Goals and Objectives of Basic Medical Education, *http://www.amc.org.au/accredgoals.asp* Accessed 26.8.01.

Bambas A. (1996). *Getting started: a survey of medical student activism*. JAMA, 276, 1436-7.

Bauman KA, Hale FA. (1985). *Bringing the homosexual patient out: Teaching the doctor's role*. Medical Education, 19, 459-62.

Berkman CS, Zinberg G. (1997). *Homophobia and heterosexism in social workers*. Social Work, 42(4), 319-30.

Bewley SJ, Bolton JGF. (1999). *Gay and lesbian issues in medical and dental education: a survey of British medical and dental schools*. MS JAMA-Report Oct 6.

Bradford J, Ryan C, Rothblum ED. (1994). *National lesbian health care survey. Implications for mental health*. J Consult Clin Psychol, 62(2), 228-42.

Brogan DJ, Frank E, Elon L, Sivanesan SP, O'Hanlan KA. (1999). *Harassment of lesbians as medical students and physicians*. MS JAMA, 282, 1290-92.

Brown R. (July 2000). *More than lip service–the report of the lesbian health information project. Royal Women's Hospital*, Victoria.

Burke BP, White JC. (2001). *Wellbeing of gay, lesbian and bisexual doctors*. BMJ, 322, 422-5.

Carroll NM. (1999). *Optimal gynaecological and obstetric care for lesbians*. Obstet Gynaecol, 93, 611-3.

Council on Scientific Affairs, AMA. (1996). *Health care needs of gay men and lesbians in the USA*. JAMA, 275, 1354-9.

Department of Human Services, South Australia. (2000). *Women's Health and Wellbeing Consultation Paper*, Adelaide.

Gay and Lesbian Medical Association (GLMA). (2000). Report, *Newsletter of the Association. LGBT Health Contacts Listing*. Fall, page 9.

Harrison AE. (1996). *Primary care of lesbian and gay patients: educating ourselves and our students*. Family Med., 28(1), 10-23.

Harrison J. (1999). *A lavender pink grey power: gay and lesbian gerontology in Australia*. Australasian Journal on Aging, Feb, 32-7.

Horsley P, Tremellen S. (1996). *Legitimising lesbian health–challenging the lack of demonstrated need argument*. Healthsharing women newsletter, 6(4), 8-11 (*Presented at the Third National Women's Health Conference*, Canberra, Nov 1995).

Johnson MH, Henderson P. (2000). *Acquiring and demonstrating attitudes in medical education: attitudes to homosexuality as a case study.* Medical Teacher, 22(6), 585-91.

King M. (1994). *Doctors and homosexuality: doctors want to know more.* BMJ, 308, 854.

Lehmann JB, Lehmann CU, Kelly PJ. (1998). *Development and health care needs of lesbians.* J Women's Health, 7(3), 379-87.

Mathews, Booth, Turner, Kessler. (1986). *Physician's attitudes toward homosexuality: a survey of a Californian medical society.* West J Med, 144, 106-10.

Mathieson CM. (1998). *Lesbian and bisexual health care. Straight talk about experiences with physicians.* Canadian Family Physician, 44, 1634-40.

McNair RP, Anderson S, Mitchell A. (2001). *Health inequalities for lesbian, gay, bisexual and transgender people: breaching the gaps, reaching the agenda.* Health Promotion J of Australia, 11(4), 305-11.

McNair RP. (2000). *Lesbian sexuality. Do GPs contribute to lesbian invisibility and ill health?* Australian Family Physician, 29(6), 514-6.

Moran N. (1996). *Lesbian health care needs.* Canadian Family Physician, 42, 879-84.

Murnane A, Smith A, Crompton L, Snow P, Munro G. (June 2000). Beyond perceptions: A report on alcohol and other drug use among gay, lesbian, bisexual and queer communities in Victoria. The ALSO Foundation, Australian Drug Foundation, Vic Health.

Northridge ME. (2001). Editor's Note: *Advancing lesbian, gay, bisexual and transgender health.* American J Public Health, 91(6), 855-6.

Oriel KA, Madlon-Kay DJ, Govaker D, Mersy D. (1996). *Gay and lesbian physicians in training: family practice program directors' attitudes and students' perceptions of bias.* Family Medicine, 28, 720-5.

Ramos MM, Tellez CM, Palley TB, Umland BE, Skipper BJ. (1998). *Attitudes of physicians practicing in New Mexico toward gay men and lesbians in the profession.* Academic Medicine, 73(4), 436-8.

Rankow EJ. (1995). *Breast and cervical cancer among lesbians.* The Jacobs Institute of Women's Health, Women's Health Issues, 5(3), 123-9.

Risdon C, Cook D, Willms D. (2000). *Gay and lesbian physicians in training: a qualitative study.* Canadian Medical Association Journal, 162(3), 331-4.

Robb N. (1996a). *Fear of ostracism still silences some gay MDs, students.* Can Med Assoc J, 155(7), 972-7.

Robb N. (1996b). *Medical schools seek to overcome 'invisibility' of gay patients, gay issues in curriculum.* Can Med Assoc J, 155(6), 765-70.

Robinson G, Cohen M. (1996). *Gay, lesbian and bisexual health care issues and medical curricula.* Can Med Assoc J, 155(6), 709-11.

Rose L. (1994). *Homophobia among doctors.* British Medical Journal, 308(6928): 586-7.

Saphira M, Glover M. (2000). *New Zealand national lesbian health survey.* Journal of Gay and Lesbian Medical Association, 4(2), 49-56.

Saunders D, Oxley J, Harvey D. (2000). *The medical profession has a reputation for conservatism, so does being gay impede your career?* BMJ, 320, S2-7233 (19 Feb).

Saunders D. (2001). *Commentary: the medical profession should face up to its own homophobia.* BMJ, 322, 424-5.

Schatz B, O'Hanlan K. (1994). Anti-Gay Discrimination in Medicine: Results of a National Survey of Lesbian, Gay and Bisexual Physicians. San Francisco: American Association of Physicians for Human Rights.

Simpson LA. (1997). *History of gay and lesbian physician groups.* J of Gay and Lesbian Medical Association, 1(1), 61-3

Smith EM, Johnson SR, Guenther SM. (1985). *Health care attitudes and experiences during gynaecological care among lesbians and bisexuals.* Am J Public Health, 75, 1085-7.

Solarz AL (editor). (1999). *Committee on Lesbian Health Research Priorities, the Institute of Medicine. Lesbian Health: Current Assessment and Directions for the Future.* Washington, DC: National Academy Press.

Stevens PE. (1995). *Structural and interpersonal impact of heterosexual assumptions on lesbian health care clients.* Nursing Research, 44(1), 25-30.

Tesar CM, Rovi SLD. (1998). *Survey of curriculum on homosexuality/bisexuality in departments of family medicine.* Family Medicine, 30(4), 283-7.

The Royal Australian College of General Practitioners. (1999). *Training program curriculum,* second edition, RACGP.

Tinmouth J, Hamwi G. (1994). *The experience of gay and lesbian medical students in medical school.* JAMA, 271(9), 714-5.

Townsend MH, Wallick MM, Cambre KM. (1991). *Support services for homosexual students at US medical schools.* Academic Medicine, 66(6), 361-3.

Townsend MH, Wallick MM, Cambre KM. (1996). *Follow up survey of support services for lesbian, gay and bisexual medical students.* Academic Medicine, 71, 1012-4.

Trippet SE, Bain J. (1992). *Reasons American lesbians fail to seek traditional health care.* Health Care for Women International, 13, 145-53.

U.S. Department of Health and Human Services (USDHHS) (2000). *Healthy People 2010.* 2nd ed. With Understanding and Improving Health and Objectives for Improving Health. 2 vols. Washington, DC: U.S. Government Printing Office, November.

Victorian Gay and Lesbian Rights Lobby. (June 2000). *Enough is enough. A report on discrimination and abuse experienced by lesbians, gay men, bisexuals and transgender people in Victoria.*

Wallick MM, Cambre KM, Townsend MH. (1992). *How the topic of homosexuality is taught at US medical schools.* Academic Medicine, 67, 601-3.

Wallick MM, Cambre KM, Townsend MH. (1995). *Influence of a freshman-year panel presentation on medical students' attitudes toward homosexuality.* Academic Medicine, 70(9), 839-41.

White JC, Dull VT. (1997). *Health risk factors and health-seeking behaviour in lesbians.* J Women's Health, 6(1), 103-12.

Not Only What You Do,
But How You Do It:
Working with Health Care Practitioners
on Gender Equality

Sharon Fonn, MBBCh, FFCH, PhD

SUMMARY. The Women's Health Project, School of Public Health, Johannesburg, South Africa, has for more than the past decade been running various gender and health training courses for participants from at least 20 different countries. In this paper I interrogate the motivation behind and methods of the gender training and offer three prompts that assist facilitators in promoting participants' understanding of gender theory. (1) Does this program/action take gender into account? (2) Does this pro-

Sharon Fonn is Associate Professor, School of Public Health, University of the Witwatersrand. She was Research Director at the Women's Health Project and engaged primarily in health systems research, health service interventions and evaluation in the public health care system in South Africa.

Address correspondence to: Professor Sharon Fonn, School of Public Health, University of the Witwatersrand, 7 York Road, Parktown 2193, Johannesburg, South Africa (E-mail: sfonn@sn.apc.org).

Much of the work described in this article is the product of a joint endeavour by colleagues at the Women's Health Project and the people involved in the project which resulted in the publication of *Transforming Health Systems: Gender and Rights in Reproductive Health.* The author would specifically like to thank Sundari Ravindran for assisting in clarifying her thoughts and Lynne Slonimsky and Barabara Klugman for commenting on early drafts.

[Haworth co-indexing entry note]: "Not Only What You Do, But How You Do It: Working with Health Care Practitioners on Gender Equality." Fonn, Sharon. Co-published simultaneously in *Women & Health* (The Haworth Medical Press, an imprint of The Haworth Press, Inc.) Vol. 37, No. 4, 2003, pp. 105-120; and: *Teaching Gender, Teaching Women's Health: Case Studies in Medical and Health Science Education* (ed: Lenore Manderson) The Haworth Medical Press, an imprint of The Haworth Press, Inc., 2003, pp. 105-120. Single or multiple copies of this article are available for a fee from The Haworth Document Delivery Service [1-800-HAWORTH, 9:00 a.m. - 5:00 p.m. (EST). E-mail address: docdelivery@haworthpress.com].

gram/action challenge gender norms? (3) Does this program/action promote women's autonomy? Examples of training sessions are described to
illustrate how our methods iterate with the content of the courses and, in
particular, how the training links to actions practitioners may engage in
to redress gender inequalities at work. I go on to argue that both structural and inter-relational aspects of health programs are important in addressing gender and health concerns and discuss the impact of such
training on participants and health services. *[Article copies available for a
fee from The Haworth Document Delivery Service: 1-800-HAWORTH. E-mail
address: <docdelivery@haworthpress.com> Website: <http://www.HaworthPress.
com> © 2003 by The Haworth Press, Inc. All rights reserved.]*

KEYWORDS. Gender equity, gender training, health worker training,
participatory methods, health service development, rights training, quality of care

Women's Health Project (WHP) is an independently funded unit in the
School of Public Health at the University of the Witwatersrand, Johannesburg,
South Africa. It articulates its mission as "working towards a society in which
there is a human rights culture and equality between women and men and conditions exist which enable women to make decisions about their lives and to
enjoy their optimum level of health." Within this brief, for about the past 10
years the organization has worked at a grassroots level, with health care planners and providers and with policy makers both nationally and internationally.
In order to achieve its mission, WHP has run a range of gender and health
courses with a variety of target groups, but significantly with practitioners involved in funding, planning and/or delivering health and development programs or services. In this article, I describe the training and our evolved
understanding of it.

Three factors motivated the WHP training approach. Firstly, the mission of
WHP seeks societal transformation, where there are shifts in social norms
(e.g., a change in the way in which men and women engage in sexual relationships so that they are satisfying and safe) rather than adhoc responses to particular health problems (e.g., promoting condoms to deal with HIV). Secondly,
there is a commitment to a specific approach to adult education which consciously engages with the notion of transformation (Freire 1970, Hope and
Timmel 1984, Haaland and Vlassoff 2001). Lastly, the background and needs
of the participants of our courses, practitioners rather than academics, led us to
develop numerous courses using teaching methods that are unconventional
compared to many university-based courses. In this article the method of training is interrogated.

I begin by attesting why training on gender inequality for this target group is required, and locate training on gender inequality within the need to train more broadly on the political economy of health. Our teaching methods are highly facilitator dependant and our training-of-trainers courses have forced us to make our facilitation methods overt. Retrospection of our methods has crystallised three questions that are useful prompts to introduce participants to gender theory. These questions and how they link to gender theory are described and discussed. As with all training courses, the content and methods iterate. I describe a few examples of activities used in our training, and explain how these both explore gender inequality and health and encourage participants to think of how they may address gender inequality in their day-to-day work. I conclude with a discussion on the impact of the courses, and how this methodological approach to training is appropriate to the audience it serves and to achieving greater awareness of and ability to impact on gender inequity in health programming.

Health status and health seeking behavior are influenced by numerous factors. These include: national economic prosperity and the priorities that are considered important in how that wealth is spent, class, race, religion, caste, age, gender, and geographic locale. These factors and other determinants interrelate (Doyal 1979). While gender is neither the sole nor often the pre-eminent determinant of health and reproductive health, exploring reproductive health through a gender lens lays bear some of the fundamental manifestations of gender inequality. Here, the issue of women's right to control their own bodies, women's right to choice, and right to autonomy of action is writ large. Women's lack of autonomy is most baldly expressed in relation to whether, how and when to have sex and children. The inability to make these decisions may affect their lives in terms of physical and psychological health and their ability to fulfil personal aspirations, whether in relation to work, economic security or leisure. Women's lack of control over their person takes many forms, from limited control over resources and ability to make independent decisions, ability to move freely in a society, and constraints due to religious mores and fear of violence.

The consequences of women's inability to exercise their sexual and reproductive rights is profound (Doyal 1998). It is seen in its most extreme form and in epidemic proportions in the excesses of preventable maternal mortality in Africa and Asia (WHO 1996). In such situations, the low status accorded to women, reflected in the absence of adequate ante-natal and delivery services means that women die as a consequence of childbirth. This is often in a social context where women's sole right to decide if they want to become pregnant is not guaranteed–choices are made on their behalf which could result in their death. The high rates of HIV infection is another example where women's status may lead them to engage in sex work, or to provide sex in exchange for school fees, or are unable to negotiate safe sex and condom use, contributing significantly to the current HIV epidemic (UNAIDS 2000). The links between socio-economic status including gender and health are well known and well documented, yet teaching of health care planners and providers rarely focuses on these social determinants of health.

Recently the contribution of gender inequality as a determinant of health and the need to take this into account in health care planning and services has been recognised. Numerous interventions have taken gender inequality into account in priority setting for development activities, in approaches to health systems management and service delivery (March 1996, Kuga Thas et al. 1996, Schalkwyk 1997, DFID 1999). The notion of mainstreaming, incorporating gender awareness within programs, is current. Translating policy into action to make a difference on the ground, at the service delivery point, is complex and difficult to achieve, however. As a result of the inadequate training of health care professionals, the people expected to take account of gender in health programming are not experts in gender analysis, and those brought in to assist are not experts in health and health services. Thus interventions are frequently semantic rather than real. To address this, people who are involved in service planning and service delivery must begin to uncover the interrelated determinants of health and their own place within it.

COURSES AND COURSE PARTICIPANTS

It is with this background in mind that the WHP has, over the past 9 years, been running courses on gender and health. The target of this training has been health care practitioners at the policy and planning level and at the provider-client interface, and has included primary care practitioners as well as managers (clinic supervisors, program managers) who support primary care delivery. Course participants come from the government and non-governmental sectors and international agencies, and have included people from a range of countries in Africa and Asia (Klugman et al. 2001). One training course (Cottingham et al. 2001) which was an institutional collaboration between WHP, the World Health Organization and Francois-Xavier Bagnoud Centre for Health and Human Rights of the Harvard School of Public Health, has run in Argentina, China, Australia and Kenya. Our choice of this target group has been deliberate and is informed by a belief that people responsible for health care planning and delivery can develop and work in a way that mitigates to some extent the impact of unequal gender relations on health.

The target audience and the aims of the course have informed the content and methods, and, as with any course, these iterate. In relation to content, three points need to be made. Firstly, the courses do not focus only on gender relations. Because the aim is to produce graduates who can develop interventions or change existing practice, it is important in training to make clear that sex-specific gender roles are determined by the complex interplay of context and institutions. Other determinants such as class, race, caste, and literacy level, may be more important than gender roles and these, too, interrelate. Simplistic solutions are unlikely to have a lasting impact. Secondly, if the courses aim to produce graduates who have an action orientation, the content needs to promote this. Lastly, we were mindful of the institutions within which course graduates work, and thus institutional barriers to change needed to be addressed in the course.

Defining and meeting the diverse needs of the target audience has been challenging. Participants on our courses include people with tertiary education and university professors, primary care providers, some who also have tertiary training but many with nursing college training only. The more highly trained staff may be familiar with reading academic articles within a circumscribed field of medical science, but most participants are unfamiliar with academic discourse on gender and many are unfamiliar with critical reading of academic articles. Participants could not be expected to engage in academic work or academic debate on gender theory, but need to engage with gender analysis.

Our pedagogic approach uses praxis to assist participants to conduct gendered critiques. This approach may not extend the boundary of academic debate, or produce course graduates able to argue the merits of different gender theories, but participants are able to develop a working understanding of gender and health. Participants in the course generate much of the content themselves. This keeps them engaged and, because they are able to do the analysis themselves, they develop a working understanding of gender inequality and find the ideas accessible and relevant.

As participants are not expected to be familiar with gender theory, it was necessary in designing the course to develop a way of assisting them to use a gender critique when interrogating programs and personal behaviors. This developed over time and drew on existing gender theory (Gender and Health Group 1999), but in retrospect, its facilitators, through using three prompts, promoted participants understanding of gender and health. These prompts were: *Does this program/action take gender into account? Does this program/action challenge gender norms? Does this program/action promote women's autonomy?*

How are these questions useful? By using the example of access to contraceptive services, I hope to make clear how these prompts introduce participants to aspects of gender theory. Take a scenario where women's freedom of movement is restricted. How, given the circumstance, can access be improved? Service providers or program managers may decide that the only way to improve women's access is to take the service to women: using a mobile service, a clinic in the village, or community-based distribution. The Program therefore works around constraints on women's mobility. Such an intervention has taken note of gender roles and found a way around them. The intervention has taken gender roles into account. In such a situation women have benefited–the service has met women's practical need; they now potentially have access to technology to control their fertility.

There is another scenario however. People managing such a program–at a national or local level, or within a NGO–may decide against the above options because such a program can only deliver a limited range of services, not the full range that could be provided at a clinic with trained nurses. Also it may not be financially feasible to provide services in each village, as opposed to centralised services. Such a program will have to find a strategy to overcome the norm that dictates that women may not move about freely. Lobbying local opinion leaders, and linking access to contraception to other health outcomes (decreasing maternal mortality), may be a method of getting people to buy into changing the status quo. Lobbying could be through advocacy initiatives, appealing to international agreements like ICPD, mobilizing like-minded community organizations, etc. The program may develop methods to lobby husbands, fathers, and brothers and influence them. Such a program, by gaining acceptance that women can avail themselves of a service irrespective of norms about freedom of movement, will have challenged gender norms. Getting participants to interrogate programs through these questions and through appropriate probes, a facilitator can help participants see the difference between the two approaches and can make clear how, in this latter case, both practical and strategic needs have been met. In this way, through examples and careful facilitation, participants are introduced to gender theory, which can be made overt after such a session when the terminology and theory can be described and discussed (Moser 1993, Kabeer 1994). Thus these first two prompts help participants to understand aspects of gender theory. Once the difference between taking gender into account and challenging gender norms has been made clear, the questions can be asked again and again, to get participants to tease out the impact programs may have on gender relations.

The question on promoting women's autonomy takes participants a step further. In both the scenarios described above, women's access to contraception will have been increased: in one instance, by taking account of gender inequality; in the other, by challenging gender norms. These are structural issues. However, it is also important to consider the intention behind increasing women's access to contraception. This is where the prompt *Does this promote women's autonomy?* is useful. This encourages participants to explore the logic behind programs. In relation to the example above, one intention could be to ensure that women have fewer children–a demographic imperative. Another could be to improve women's health, by increasing birth intervals and/or reducing numbers of pregnancies. Increasing women's access to contraception may also increase women's control over their bodies and their lives. Delaying childbirth may increase young women's chances of finishing school, completing tertiary education, getting jobs, and improving their economic circumstance. Clearly, this is dependant on where a woman lives. Promoting a woman's autonomy recognizes that if she lives in a situation where there is no chance of employment or economic advancement, she may choose to have a child, even at a young age, as this in and of itself may give her life meaning. Deciding when and if to have a child may give a woman a greater sense of control over her own destiny. In this case, a provider would need to support her choice not to use contraception. By asking this question participants are asked to explore the ideology underlying both programs and their own place in it.

The intention behind the service (controlling a woman's fertility, improving her health, or promoting her autonomy) will influence the nature of provider-client interaction. What the provider says and how s/he relates to individual women will be different. Where the central concern is to promote women's autonomy, the range of contraceptive choices available, and the option of using none, would have to be offered with sufficient information to allow an individual to decide. A provider needs to determine if there are any absolute contraindications and then inform the woman about how one takes the method, how much it interferes with one's usual day-to-day life, and the range of potential side effects. Locating this technical information contextually for an individual woman is required to promote her sense of individual autonomy. Thus a discussion between provider and client needs to pay attention to personal priorities: How will decisions taken now influence the future, and how will a choice make a woman feel? Often the question of promoting women's autonomy brings participants to challenge their own beliefs. For example, if you are employed to run a contraception service, then you may believe (perhaps subconsciously) that all women who come to your service should leave with a contraceptive. This belief is reinforced by target-driven monitoring of services. Frequently, providers and planners have difficulty in accepting that for women with few choices in life, having a child, even at an early age or with other children, may give meaning to a woman's life. Thus the question regarding women's autonomy begins to explore the roles of individuals' actions and behaviours within health services.

Other questions/scenarios, once presented to participants, can be interrogated through the question *Does this promote women's autonomy?* Where husbands have traditionally had primary say in choices around child bearing, promoting women's autonomy involves questioning this assumption; this may require that both the client and providers suspend their beliefs. A provider may assist women to circumvent the control of men, by maintaining confidentiality and allowing to keep her contraceptive use hidden from her partner: this is often purported to be the reason why injectable methods are so popular in sub-Saharan Africa. Thus the nature of the interaction can contribute to providing a service that promotes women's autonomy. I am arguing that both structural and relational circumstances of a service are important in addressing gender inequalities. This can be done in ways that take gender into account, challenge gender norms, and/or promote women's autonomy. These three questions are hooks that assist facilitators and participants to begin to unpack gender theory and raise the position of self within gender analysis.

HOW DO THE COURSES DEAL
WITH THIS RELATIONAL ASPECT?

It is clear from these examples that to incorporate gender equality into programming requires an understanding of the determinants of health, the interplay between these determinants and, at the provider-client interface, an understanding of self. Implicit in our methodological approach is that gender relations are premised on deeply embedded, entrenched and taken-for-granted assumptions about what it means to be a woman/man, what counts as valid ways of relating and what our rights and entitlements are as gendered beings. Gender relations are forms of consciousness which are taken-for-granted and continue as we are often unaware that we hold these assumptions and participate in these ways of behaving. One has to work with these embedded constructs–to show how we impose our own history of relationships with others onto people with whom we interact. These are not only personal ways of behaving but are common in society and institutions. These methods of relating are not value free but result in systematic inequalities that extend beyond ourselves. It is important in training to develop methods that help to explore how we relate, that we relate in particular ways that are patterned, and that these patterned ways of relating often run across different spheres in which we are involved. Resources for reflecting are required that enable participants to see themselves in new ways and to imagine new ways of relating. To achieve this, it is essential that the training includes methods of self-reflection.

The methodologies we use are participatory and demand that participants actively generate and discuss the content of the course. The skeleton, the process, and the learning activities are prescribed, but the content is generated through the learning process. Participants are given an opportunity to reassess their usual practice from a point of view that locates their clients as well as themselves in their social and economic context. Specific prompts lay bare gender relations. Participants use examples from their everyday experience, their own worldview, rather than a theoretical base. The methods used are well known and described in many manuals (Williams 1994, Hope, Hartigan et al.

1997), and we have drawn on these and developed them further. We use simulation games and role-plays, case histories, poetry, songs, local idioms, and structured exercises.

How does this work? A scenario–for example, a woman presenting to a clinic complaining of infertility–is presented. The aim is to get participants to express how they make sense of the scenario, to elicit their taken-for-granted constructs so that they can be opened up for discussion. Participants are prompted to answer the question why the woman is infertile. Once that is answered–for example, she has an untreated sexually transmitted disease–they have to answer why this is untreated. For each answer, the participants have to question why this is the case. Participants thus build a matrix of why this woman is in this situation. They physically build their argument on a sheet of paper. Responses include that the woman did not seek treatment for a previous reproductive tract inflection. If left at this point, the women herself is constructed as at fault. However, the process forces participants to ask why did she not get treatment. This opens up a range of possibilities: no service; a service without drugs to provide treatment; a service that is hostile; she did not know how to interpret her symptoms; she had no money to access services; her partner was not able to talk to her when he had a sexually transmitted disease so that she was not treated when he was treated. Now the woman is not at fault; providers have located her in her social and economic context. As the participants generate this list themselves, the reasons why providers think a patient may be infertile are likely to bear a close relationship to locally specific problems, whether reflecting facts or interpretations. Either way this is useful material to work with. Once the chain of causation is analysed we ask participants to look at each link in the chain and develop potential interventions. Once a fuller analysis has been undertaken, interventions suggest themselves. Access to services can be increased, drug supply systems improved, or provider hostility towards clients resolved. Education for women on RTIs, economic self-sufficiency, promoting notions of joint accountability for reproductive health and male responsibility, are possible areas of intervention. Not only has a more detailed analysis of the problem been achieved, but a link to action is being developed.

Through such activities, participants are able to explore how they construct health, treatment, women, and the way of the world. The explanations paradigm is not unidimensional. Issues of race, class, gender and geography, and factors acting at household, community and national level, are explored. Not one determinant, but the matrix, is explored, and this is the case in each activity. The aim is to expose the entire interlinking matrix. The role of the facilitator is to make these links clear and to make the connection between participants' choices and gender theory. The activities reinforce how gender operates within the broader context, and in this way, the content iterates with the methods.

One activity called the spider-web (Cottingham 2001) presents a case history of an individual and participants interact by answering questions about this case history. At each point in this woman's life, when a particular event has occurred, participants are asked, from a predetermined set of options (sex, gender, politics, economics, culture) for the underlying explanation for her circumstance. For example, a woman may have had a child at 14 years of age. Participants have to consider why this is so. Some will say the basis for understanding this is culture–women marry young. Others will say that it reflects the low status of women and lack of access to education, but that it is not culture but gender. Others may say it is because there is no employment and having a child is the only meaningful activity open to young girls–hence it is an economic issue. Participants choose to take a stand physically, with areas of the floor labelled culture, gender, economics, politics, etc., and literally build a web by passing a ball of string from participant to participant as each person categorises the underlying reason for particular outcomes in the case study. Conflicting analyses, as long as they are well motivated, are allowed. So for one outcome numerous explanations are possible. The notion of the complex web of causality is generated by them and is physically re-enforced by the activity.

One exercise uses a method of discourse analysis. Participants are asked to free-associate in relation to specific health education materials. In doing so, they again lay bare preconceived ideas they–and the people developing the materials–hold. In this exercise, participants deconstruct assumptions and build alternative messages that may be less victim blaming, for example, or may promote male responsibility for sexual behavior. Again the three questions described above are useful prompts. One example used is a poster from a Mozambican government education campaign on sexually transmitted infections (STIs). The poster depicts couples going to a STI treatment centre. In the discussion, participants said that the poster promotes the idea that both members of a couple are involved in and responsible for reproductive health and that they can deal with the issue together. Participants felt that the poster promoted the idea of joint responsibility for sexual health and thus challenged gender norms and promoted women's autonomy. An interesting talking point from this particular poster was the depiction of an elderly couple going to the STI clinic. Initially participants said these people must be at the wrong clinic; through this, it was possible to talk about sex and sexual satisfaction and to explore people's attitudes to age and sex. It allowed for discussion about the legitimacy of older people being sexual beings. It was possible, too, to explore prejudice about youth sexuality, and to explore how providers can be judgmental towards clients, based on their own ideas about what is acceptable or not. Useful prompts in such a situation included asking participants if their opinions change if a young person is a boy rather than a girl. Hence the poster allowed us to explore providers' assumptions about gender and age, and different attitudes to male and female sexuality. Again, this exercise draws attention to both social convention and the role we as providers or health planners play to reinforce or challenge social norms.

Role-plays are also useful. A short scenario is offered and participants develop it as they like. One role-play, used with hundreds of course participants, is a scenario of a pregnant woman who arrives at a clinic late in her labour. The actors, course participants who are health care providers themselves, develop the scene and almost invariably illustrate a situation where this woman is scolded for coming at an advanced stage in her labour. With appropriate prompts led by the facilitator, this is explored: Why is the woman late? Why is there no transport? Where is the father? This directs participants to analyse various assumptions that they have about the patient, her circumstances and gender roles. In answering these questions, providers construct what they know and think about their patients from their own experience. They also have an opportunity to look at their own (blaming) behavior. Again, the link to action is developed by asking participants to suggest interventions. These have included: lobbying local politicians to build better roads, insisting that fathers come to at least one ante-natal visit, working with local chiefs to build a sense of responsibility among men for their wives' health, and being more understanding towards patients. Other examples from similar scenarios have brought forth other interventions to challenge gender norms like asking a father (rather than the mother) to bring his child to the child health clinic, and not blaming a woman for returning on the "wrong day" for repeat medications when she may have little control over her time. Again, the processes we use promote a multidimensional understanding of the social construction of health and health seeking behaviour, and encourage people to think about taking action. Further, by using role-plays (in this instance), we give providers an opportunity to be self-reflecting.

Irrespective of the content, role-plays demand that people put themselves in the position of another person, and are a powerful and fun method to build empathy. Exploring unequal gender relations is something we have all experienced, and using personal examples appears to be crucial in these courses. The similarity of personal experience and that of their clients/patients, in spite of vast differences between them, builds a sense of empathy. This motivates participants to articulate changes that might be introduced in program planning or implementation and in individual action. The method itself, as well as the content, is material to increase people's understanding of gender inequality, ability to generate interventions to deal with gender inequality, and willingness to act. Through this, drawing on their personal experience in the home, the workplace and public life, participants develop an organic understanding of the impact of gender inequality on health and on their own work organizations.

People apply principles without necessarily being fully conversant with the underlying theory or its language.

One concern of the courses is the need to engage in some way with the institutions where individuals work. This is dealt with in two ways. Firstly, in the courses we explored the idea that institutions themselves are gendered, not in a theoretical way but encouraging participants to analyse their own institutions. In the gender and health courses that we have run, participants have described how certain tasks, such as changing of diapers in paediatric wards, are simply not done by male nurses and participants admitted that prior to the course they had not thought about it. It was taken-for-granted that this was not men's work and drew attention to women's as well as men's roles in gender typing (Britton 2000). Participants also described how their organizations mirror society, with men making decisions about resources such as transport and equipment. They also noted that consequent on transformation in the South African health sector post-1994, increasingly women are in positions of authority but that this does not guarantee changes in how decisions are made or how people inter-relate. On some courses, people have spoken of the need to change policies to make institutions more woman-friendly or to give more voice to women. However, transformation is not easy (Roa et al. 1997, Rao et al. 2000).

The second manner in which the courses have taken on institutional issues is to locate gender-sensitive providers within their working environment. This has been a feature of *Health Workers for Change* (Fonn et al. 1996) and *Health Workers for Choice* (Varkey et al. 2001). These training courses aim to improve quality of care by taking a gendered health systems approach to interpersonal aspects of quality of care and focus specifically on the provider-client interface. The courses, available as manuals, explicitly state that it is essential that managers are well-informed about the course, and are ready to listen and respond to demands that this process will generate. The training also takes cognisance of the fact that there are many requirements to enable providers to deliver better quality and more gender sensitive services. This includes having a functional health care system, reliable drug supplies, available transport, less hierarchical management systems, a system that provides for the workers themselves, timely salary and overtime payment, adequate accommodation, and so on. (Fonn et al. 2001, Fonn et al. 1998).

Our training methods appear to work well with a wide range of audiences, from university professors and heads of units in hospitals to nurses in clinics and cleaners. The method depends on good facilitation, however, with someone conversant in gender analysis and health care. Much of what is explored is done through the probing of the facilitator.

Course participants have frequently noted that the potential interventions they identify are practical, small things–not what they imagine a gender program to be. Addressing or redressing gender inequality is often possible through inexpensive and small-scale changes at the provider-client interface, or changes in nuances of programs. Including men as well as women in an education program, for example, can have considerable impact. Participants state that while they have been on gender training before, this is the first time that links between analysis and action have been made overtly and appear possible.

WHAT EVIDENCE IS THERE THAT THIS METHOD OF TRAINING WORKS AND HAS AN IMPACT?

Within the sessions, it is clear how people's analysis develops. Participants also come up with feasible interventions. Evaluations of our courses are ongoing and provide positive feedback. At the personal level, the courses have had an impact. In one instance, a participant took her husband to court for assault, to which she had been subjected for years; it was only after the course that she said she was able to make it public. A six-month follow-up of participants of the WHP annual 3-week course asked participants if, consequent on the course, there had been any changes in their personal life. In the 1997 follow-up, 15 of the 30 participants replied and all said there had been changes. These included: "I push people at home to no longer follow gender stereotype roles"; "Boys are washing dishes at home, girls are chopping wood"; "My husband helps in the kitchen"; "I think about how things will affect me and my health before deciding to do them"; "I talk about these issues in my other activities like at my mothers union and church"; "I am more sensitive to women"; "I am more supportive of my female friends"; "I now read–especially on women's issues"; "I applied for a scholarship."

Course graduates also described changes they made at work that they ascribed to being on the course. While most consisted of report-back sessions about the course to colleagues, nursing schools, and workshops with providers, some also included making funds available for workshops on violence against women. People also described changes in personal behavior at work: "I treat people more on a first come, first served, basis rather than men first, and have manipulated my co-workers to do the same"; "I participate in debates more"; "Now I drive the mobile myself instead of getting a male driver." Again this reflects personal changes that do not require institutional change and are within the power of the individual. At the institutional level, change was described as difficult. It seems that a critical mass of people who are thinking in the same way is required. A number of participants noted that "other categories in the hospital and community should attend the course" and it is "hard to tell others who were not there what it is all about." Externalities, the openness of organizations to change, and the presence of a critical mass of people to support change–are factors that influence this. Further, most of the participants in our courses work within large bureaucracies and affecting change is not easy. As one participant said, "It has been hard for me as I am in a department where I cannot implement things" and that being on the course "highlighted what sterile ground we have here (at our own work)."

WHAT IS THE IMPACT ON SERVICES?

Health Workers for Change has been evaluated in a longitudinal study in a variety of settings and this indicated that it is a useful health system development tool, makes a positive contribution to quality of care from the perspective of service users (Onyango Ouma et al. 2001), and is a useful method to mainstream gender in health systems development (Vlassoff et al. 2001). A much smaller impact assessment of a similar tool to improve abortion access has also been evaluated and yielded encouraging results, indicating that this kind of training, to make people aware of the gender and socio-economic determinants of unwanted pregnancy, can change providers' attitudes to the provision of abortion services (Varkey et al. 2000).

We conclude that this pedagogic approach, working with people's own constructs, can increase understanding, assist participants to develop interventions, and build motivation to act to decrease gender inequalities. These are bounded by the environment in which individuals operate. The gendered nature of institutions and societies means that while gender training has a place and can impact at the interpersonal level and to some extent within health care provision, it is not a panacea. However, for this target audience, practitioners in health and development programs, we have a methodology that assists both planners and providers to come to grips with theory and apply it in their work.

REFERENCES

Britton, D.M. (2000). *The epistemology of the gendered organization*. Gender and Society 14(3):418-434.

Cottingham, J., Fonn, S., Gruskin, S., Klugman, B., Moreno, C., Mwau, A., Ravindran, S., Snow, R., Xaba, M. (2001). *Transforming health systems: gender and rights in reproductive health*. A training curriculum for health programme managers. Geneva, World Health Organization.

Department for International Development, United Kingdom (1999). Department for International Development, *Gender Equality Mainstreaming (GEM) Information Resource*. DFID Intranet, draft 2001.

Doyal, L., and the WHO Working Group on Gender (1998). *Gender and Health Technical Paper, Women's Health and Development*. World Health Organization.

Fonn, S., Xaba M. (1996). *Health Workers for Change.* WHP/WHO Geneva.

Fonn, S., Xaba, M., Tint, K., Conco, D., Varkey S. (1998). *Maternal health services in South Africa.* South African Medical Journal 88:697-702.

Fonn, S., Mtonga, A., Nkoloma, H., Kyomuhendo, G., Asiimwe, F., daSilva, L., Kazilimani, E., Davis, S., Dia, R. (2001). *Health providers opinions on provider-client relations: Results of a multi-country study to test health workers for change.* Health Policy and Planning 16(Suppl.1):19-23.

Freire, P. (1970). *Pedagogy of the oppressed.* New York: Continuum.

Gender and Health Group, Liverpool School of Tropical Medicine (1999). *Guidelines for the Analysis of Gender and Health.* Liverpool School of Tropical Medicine and Department for International Development, United Kingdom.

Haaland, A., Vlassoff, C. (2001). *Introducing health workers for change: From transformation theory to health systems in developing countries.* Health Policy and Planning 16(suppl.1):1-6.

Hartigan, P., Gomez, E., da Silva, J., de Schutter, M. (1997). *Workshop on Gender, Health and Development: Facilitator's Guide.* Pan American Health Organization (PAHO), Washington, DC.

Hope, A., Timmel, S. (1984). *Training for Transformation* Volumes 1, 2 and 3. Mambo Press, Harare.

Kabeer, N. (1994). *Reversed Realities: Gender Hierarchies in Development Thought.* Verso, London.

Klugman, B., Fonn, S., Tint, K. (2001). *Reproductive Health for All.* AIDOS, Italy and Women's Health Project, South Africa.

Kuga Thas, A., Surgey, D., Abdullah, R. (1996). *Women-Centred and Gender-Sensitive Experiences: Changing Our Perspectives, Policies and Programmes on Women's Health in Asia and the Pacific: Health Resource Kit.* Kuala Lumpur, Asian-Pacific Resource and Research Centre for Women (ARROW).

March, C. (1996). *A Tool Kit: Concepts and Frameworks for Gender Analysis and Planning.* Oxfam UK/Ireland, Oxford.

Moser, M. (1993). *Gender Planning and Development: Theory, Practice and Training.* Routledge, London.

Onyango Ouma, W., Laisser, R., Mbilima, M., Araoye, M., Pittman, P., Agyepong, I., Zakari, M., Fonn, S., Tanner, M., Vlassoff, C. (2001). *An evaluation of health workers for change in seven settings: A useful management and health system development tool.* Health Policy and Planning 16(Suppl.1):24-32.

Rao, A., Stuart, R. (1997). *Rethinking organizations: A feminist perspective.* Gender and Development 5(1):10-16.

Rao, A., Kelleher, D. (2000). *Leadership for social transformation: Some ideas and questions on institutions and feminist leadership.* Gender and Development 8(3): 74-79.

Schalkwyk, J., Woroniuk, B., Thomas, H., in close consultation with the Health Division and the Gender Equality Unit at Sida (1997). *Handbook for Mainstreaming. A Gender Perspective in the Health Sector.* Department for Democracy and Social Development, Health Division, Sida-Swedish International Development Cooperation Agency, Stockholm.

Varkey, S., Fonn, S., Ketlhapile, M. (2000). *The role of advocacy in implementing the South African abortion law*. Reproductive Health Matters 8(16):103-111.

Varkey, S., Fonn, S., Ketlhapile, M. (2001). *Health Workers for Choice*. Women's Health Project. Johannesburg.

Vlassoff, C., Fonn, S. (2001). *Health workers for change as a health systems management and development tool*. Health Policy and Planning 16(Suppl.1):47-52.

Williams, S. with Seed, J., Mwau, A. (1994). *The Oxfam Gender Training Manual*. Oxfam. Oxford.

The Integration of Gender in Medical Research and Education– Obstacles and Possibilities from a Nordic Perspective

Anne Hammarström, MD, PhD

SUMMARY. Research on women's issues in medicine was developed in the Nordic countries from the beginning of the 1980s. The theoretical developments led to a change of concepts from women's health to gender research, within which the structurally organised relations between men and women are analysed. Over the last decades, gender research has slowly been established in medical faculties, as a result of a strong political commitment for increased research and integration of gender issues in the university curriculum in Sweden. The government has made substantial investments in order to stimulate gender research and education in different disciplines, with special focus on medicine. Academic medicine has responded to this development with different strategies, including resistance and redefining concepts. Gender research has slowly become integrated into both research and teaching within Nordic academic medicine, although the pathway has not been easy. Gender research has had political support but there is a risk of backlash.

Anne Hammarström is affiliated with the Department of Public Health and Clinical Medicine, Division of Family Medicine, Umeå University, S-901 85 Umeå, Sweden (E-mail: anne.hammarstrom@fammed.umu.se).

[Haworth co-indexing entry note]: "The Integration of Gender in Medical Research and Education–Obstacles and Possibilities from a Nordic Perspective." Hammarström, Anne. Co-published simultaneously in *Women & Health* (The Haworth Medical Press, an imprint of The Haworth Press, Inc.) Vol. 37, No. 4, 2003, pp. 121-133; and: *Teaching Gender, Teaching Women's Health: Case Studies in Medical and Health Science Education* (ed: Lenore Manderson) The Haworth Medical Press, an imprint of The Haworth Press, Inc., 2003, pp. 121-133. Single or multiple copies of this article are available for a fee from The Haworth Document Delivery Service [1-800-HAWORTH, 9:00 a.m. - 5:00 p.m. (EST). E-mail address: docdelivery@haworthpress.com].

Medical students' reactions to gender education can be compared with academic medicine's reactions towards gender research. Obstacles and possibilities are described in relation to teaching gender in schools of medicine.

Most important is to recognise the risks for increased gender stereo-types and increased essentialism among the students, unless gender is taught from a theoretical perspective. *[Article copies available for a fee from The Haworth Document Delivery Service: 1-800-HAWORTH. E-mail address: <docdelivery@haworthpress.com> Website: <http://www.HaworthPress. com> © 2003 by The Haworth Press, Inc. All rights reserved.]*

KEYWORDS. Medical gender research, resistance, integration, teaching strategies

INTRODUCTION

During the last two decades, there has been strong political commitment in the Nordic countries, especially in Sweden, to increased research on gender and the integration of gender issues into the university curriculum. The Swedish Government has made significant investments to stimulate gender research and gender education. However, especially in medicine, the implementation of these resources has not been easy because of resistance from the academy. In this paper, I describe the process of integrating gender issues into medical research and education. The paper deals with the historical development as well as the impact of political investments in relation to gender, and the response of academic medicine to gender research. What happened to the government resources? How did the universities try to redefine gender so that the research resources could be used for other purposes, for example, for research on men and women rather than on gender issues? The differences between research on women and gender research will also be analysed. Finally, my experiences of teaching gender in medicine will be summarised as seven lessons learned. I also raise the question of integration of gender in the whole curriculum: Is this desirable or not?

THE DEVELOPMENT OF GENDER IN MEDICINE

From Women's Studies to Gender Research

Research on women's issues in medicine was developed in the Nordic countries from the beginning of the 1980s, in close co-operation with the international research community (Hammarström et al. 2001). The research focused on both women's health issues and on power inequalities between men and women. During the 1980s, theoretical developments led to a change of concepts from women's research to gender research, with a focus on structurally organised relations between men and women. The concept of "women's studies," however, is still being used by some researchers in the Nordic countries, especially in Finland. In contrast, the concept of "feminism" dominates the Anglo-American research, and this is increasingly being used in all Nordic countries. Both gender and feminist research draw on theories about gender. However, only feminist research is also based on political action–often in close collaboration with the women's movement–as well as social change (Hammarström 1999). Therefore, feminist research is useful in public health, especially in health promotion. In this paper, I use "gender," as this is the term used by Swedish authorities when discussing integration.

The terms "sex" and "gender" are often used synonymously in medicine although they have fundamentally different meanings. While "sex" refers to the biological differences between men and women (e.g., chromosomes, internal and external sex organs, hormonal makeup and secondary sex characteristics), the term "gender" was introduced in order to separate biological sex from the social, cultural and historical construction of femininity and masculinity (Rubin 1975). Thus, gender research draws attention to the fact that differences between men and women are not constant or unimpressionable. Rather, gender refers to how men and women are interpreted in different cultures and how masculinities and femininities are shaped continuously and differently across time and space (Connell 1987, West & Zimmerman 1987). Gender is not only an individual characteristic. According to Connell (1987), relationships between men and women need to be seen as a part of a larger pattern of gender relationships in all sectors in society, the "gender order" in which male domination is created and maintained. Thus, gender relations emphasised in gender research are not primarily based on couples, but on the structurally organised relationships between men and women in society. The gender order in society is the base for its gendered division of work (both waged and domestic), resources and power. In the labour market, for example, occupations become gendered as they are characterized by qualities, attributes and behaviours assigned to men or women, respectively.

Before the term "gender" came into use, the term "sex" was applied to gender differences whether they were biological, social or cultural. Biological differences were regarded as original and naturally occurring differences between men and women, and were considered to be of primary importance. Biology was, and still is, treated in conventional medical research as unchangeable and deterministic, as well as the actual cause of a number of social and psychological differences between women and men. Gender researchers in medicine have criticised the stark distinction made between immutable biological sex, on the one hand, and social/cultural constructed gender on the other (Hammarström et al. 2001). Biological and social factors should be analysed simultaneously; what is considered "biological" may also be socially determined, and vice versa. The need to analyse the interplay between sex and gender is of special importance in medicine (where biological factors obviously are of importance), compared to gender research in other disciplines.

Why Gender Research Rather Than Research on Women's Health?

What can a gender perspective contribute within medicine? Why is it important to use a gender theoretical analysis rather than to focus on women's health? First of all, research focusing on empirical descriptions of women's (and men's) health without any interpretation of the findings increases the risk for essentialism, that is, the tendency to regard differences between men and women as constant, general and unimpressionable. For example, in a qualitative analysis of medical articles which focused gender differences in revascularisation of patients' with coronary heart disease, the explanatory models for the gender differences were analysed (Löfmark & Hammarström 2001). Although the articles stated that they focused on gender differences, our analysis showed that there was almost no discussion of the results with regard to gender. When a possible explanation was mentioned, the authors mostly referred to biological or psychological differences between men and women.

Different methods can be used in order to diminish the risk of over-generalisation of gender differences. One way is to make the differences among women (and among men) visible, with regard to class, race, ethnicity, age, sexual orientation, religion, and so on. Often these differences are larger than the differences between men and women (MacIntyre et al. 1996). The most important way to diminish essentialism is to interpret the findings in a gender framework. Gender research starts where other research ends, analysing the findings from a gender theoretical perspective (Hammarström 1999).

Second, focusing on women's issues often leaves men and masculinity out of the analysis. Thus, it seems as if women–in contrast to men–are considered to have a gender, while men are regarded as the sexless and the genderless norm.

Third, gender research has many changing potentials compared to research on women's and men's health. The changing potentials of gender research can be summarised as follows (Hammarström 1999): (1) New research areas are identified, based on gendered questions such as the importance of the male norm, gendered life circumstances and gendered expressions of health. (2) Power differences are exposed and analysed, e.g., violence against women at the level of interpersonal relationships, and policies towards gender-based violence at the state level. (3) Gender theories contribute to understanding gendered phenomena in health, e.g., the impact of gender constructions on health (Connell 2000, Courtney 2000), the normalisation of sexual violence (Lundgren 1995), or the gendered rehabilitation process (Ahlgren & Hammarström 1999).

From the Periphery to the Centre

From the beginning, gender research in medicine in the Nordic countries was performed by a network of researchers on the periphery, outside the establishment. Over time, gender research has slowly been established in medical faculties, especially in Sweden and Norway. This has not been an easy process as academic medicine in has been resistant to this (Hammarström 2002). In Norway, the process was easier as the Medical Research Council supported the integration of gender into medical research. Medical gender research in the Nordic countries can now be described as a scientific research area, with academic positions, around twenty published academic theses, and several doctoral students currently enrolled. National, Nordic and international conferences have been held and around seven special journal issues have been published within the field. The latest was an international special issue on feminism in public health (Hammarström 1999). Gender is no longer on the periphery, but is moving into the middle of the medical nucleus.

In the section that follows, I will concentrate on the Swedish experiences, where gender has been more integrated in academic medicine compared to the other Nordic countries. Before that, I will briefly mention some of the background to the resistance towards gender in the medical academy.

The historical development shows that Swedish medicine today has its roots in two patriarchal traditions: academic medicine with its closeness to church, and practical surgery with its close ties to the military (Gustafsson 1987). Over time, a pattern emerged: The medics with their academic education had control over many disciplines, while the barber-surgeons, with their connection to military power, continued their practical work without scientific basis. History shows that part of the medical practice lacked scientific connection. Restricted scientific bases are still obvious in certain parts of today's medicine and in medical education. Compared to other field of academic education, medical education for a long time lacked scientific training, research preparation, and analytic points of departure. A great deal of clinical practice is still based on trial and error rather than on evidence-based medicine. Medical education has been criticised for still being dominated by ideas from 17th century Cartesianism, e.g., in relation to the separation of body and mind (Burger 2001). This separation has been facilitated by the exceptional position of positivism in medicine, as early as 1910 when the Flexner Report presented guidelines in the US for how positivistic ways of thinking should permeate the whole medical education (Berliner 1975). Western medicine today is still largely dominated by a positivistic standpoint, which holds the belief that there is one true explanation to illnesses and this explanation can often be measured and judged in an objective way. Positivism is so taken for granted that it is not always experienced as a theory, but rather as a matter of fact.

Political Investments

The political arena has had a considerable influence on the institutionalisation of gender research in academic medicine. A prerequisite for the political interest has been the close collaboration between medical gender researchers, women's political organisations, and the women's movement. Medical gender research has developed in close collaboration with the women's movement, for example, organisations providing for women who are subject to violence. Within political parties in Sweden (especially the Social Democrats, the Left Party and the Liberal Party), women have been engaged in supporting gender research, in particular in medicine. Several times, women's political organisations from all parliamentary parties have joined together to propose investments in gender research. These organisations have functioned as pressure groups on the government, and their lobbying has resulted in important decisions regarding financial resources. This financial support since the mid 1980s has been a precondition for the development of gender research within academic medicine. However, most of these investments have been isolated measures. In order for gender research to further develop, policies need to be changed so that these investments are built into the structures rather than gender researchers being dependent on political trends.

I have argued so far that academic medicine has been under pressure to accept gender research from above (the political arena) and from below (gender researchers within the field). Next, the response of academic medicine is described.

ACADEMIC MEDICINE– RESISTANCE AND THE POWER TO DEFINE

How Are Governmental Priorities Transformed?

In recent years, political investments and priorities within the field of gender in medicine have been willingly embraced by academic medicine. Despite this, representatives from the medical faculties have tried to transform the resources and shift the focus from gender to research on women (and men). How this process takes place can be illustrated with the appointment of the first professorship in medical women's studies, which constituted a part of the Swedish Government's political investment in the field (Hammarström 2002). In the advertisement for the position, women's studies were defined as a research area, dealing with the connection between women's health and women's life circumstances. Three reviewers were appointed, none of whom had qualifications in the field. Only one of the reviewers defined how she evaluated the applicants' overall qualifications (Reviewers' opinion 1993): she used six criteria, of which one was related to competence within the field of women's studies (women's position, life circumstances). Each criterion was worth one point, and hence the reviewer had reduced the applicants' competence within women's studies to a single criterion. Beyond that, she speculated that the basic biological research performed by one applicant (later recommended for the position) could have *implications* for women's life circumstances, and by doing so, women's studies were transformed to include any research that might possibly have implications for women's life circumstances. Later, she stated that she preferred biological explanations to any power-related explanatory model to explain or account for gender differences in mortality. Thus, this 'scientific evaluation' was built on the reviewer's personal interpretation of the field and her personal dislike of power models. The example illustrates how representatives from academic medicine can transform women's studies into any biological research on women.

The appointment of the first professorship in gender studies at another medical faculty underwent a similar process. As the appointment concerned me, I will only briefly mention that the medical faculty tried to disregard the reviewers' recommendations. The reason expressed unofficially was that my research belonged to social science and not to medicine, because it focused on theory and power analysis. Eventually, I won the appeal on the basis of my superior qualifications in gender research. The story is one example of the role of central authorities in the institutionalisation of gender in medicine.

The Scandal of the Medical Research Council

In 1995, the board of the Swedish Medical Research Council (MRC) was dismissed. One contributory cause was the sharp criticism of their gendered distribution of funding (Wold & Wennerås 1997). Two medical doctors, Agnes Wold and Christine Wennerås, as had several other women, applied for research funding, but were unsuccessful. When they asked for all peer-review scores, the MRC officials initially refused them access to the documents. However, the Swedish Freedom of the Press Act guarantees all individuals free access to all documents held by state or municipal authorities and thus, the MRC was forced to release their scores. Wold and Wennerås analysed the scores for 114 applicants for 20 postdoctoral fellowships (65 men and 52 women) and found that the women were given lower average scores than the men on all three evaluation parameters (scientific competence, quality of proposed methodology, relevance of the research proposal). The women applicants were deemed particularly deficient in scientific competence. Therefore, Wold and Wennerås analysed the scientific productivity of each applicant in different ways (total number of original scientific publications, number of first author articles, the impact factor of the journal, science citation database, etc.). Their conclusion was that two factors had a significant influence on peer review ratings of scientific competence. The first was the gender of the applicant: in order to receive the same competence score as the men, women had to be 2.5 times more productive than the average male applicant. The second was the affiliation of the applicant with a committee member; the affiliation bonus was of the same magnitude as the 'male gender' bonus.

The new committee in MRC (as well as the newly established Scientific Council of Medicine (SCM) within The Swedish Research Council which now replaces the MRC) made an effort to share their research grants more equally between men and women. So the criticism had a great impact on the gendered distribution of funding. However, so far few research projects on gender research have been financed. Medical gender researchers are instead referred to a special committee on gender research for all disciplines. This committee has around 10 million Swedish crowns (SEK) (1 SEK = US$ 0.13) to distribute on gender research in the humanities, social science, natural science and medicine per annum, compared to the around 400 million SEK that SCM has primarily for basic medical research, within which gender research is totally absent. Thus, there is a lack of funding for gender studies in medicine (and in other disciplines) and more resources are needed to further develop the subject.

Because of governmental directions, the SCM decided to judge all applications in year 2003 after an old-fashioned biological definition of gender as well as to allocate a small amount of money to subjects like multi-disciplinary research and gender. No competence in gender issues is needed in order to judge these applications. Thus, here is another example of how representatives from academic medicine transform gender research into any biological research on women and men.

Teaching Gender in Medicine

I have described how gender research is slowly integrating within academic medicine. The difficulties related to this process will influence the medical training of students (as discussed by Westerståhl et al. this volume). In this final section, I describe some aspects of the Swedish experience of teaching gender in medicine, and summarise the lessons learnt.

In a proposition in 1994, the Swedish Government concluded that special attention needed to be paid towards increasing knowledge about women's health in medical training. In order to stimulate teaching about women's health, the government established a special fund to which medical faculties around the country could apply. One of the projects funded was used for gender analyses of medical textbooks (Alexandersson et al. 1998). While it is obvious that the male norm is present in the course literature, few studies have evaluated medical textbooks from a gender perspective and standard instruments or protocol for such assessment is lacking. The work from Linköping University entailed the construction of an instrument to facilitate gender analysis in medical textbooks (Alexandersson 1999). A protocol with 33 questions was designed to investigate the following questions:

- To what extent is the text presented and analysed for women and men separately?
- Are gendered factors, such as life circumstances, medicalisation, attitudes, etc., taken into consideration?
- Are female-dominated diseases, illnesses and risk factors presented?
- Are the clinical methods of treatment developed and effective for both men and women?
- Is the male norm present?
- What is the implication of the gender of the author and of the physicians in the text?

By applying this protocol in nine medical textbooks in different subjects, the author showed its value in gender analysis. Gender bias (such as the male norm, less attention given to female-dominated disorders, false picture of male dominance among physicians, stereotyped gender patterns, etc.) was apparent in most of the literature. Thus, gender can not be integrated into the medical curriculum, unless medical textbooks are analysed from a gender perspective and either changed or critically discussed with the students. The analyses led to increased awareness of gender bias among teachers at the faculty. In addition, as a voluntary task, the medical students at Linköping University now have the opportunity to analyse their literature with the protocol.

Some official documents favour the inclusion of gender in the medical education. According to the Swedish Regulation of Higher Education (appendix 2, point 22), medical students must have "acquired knowledge about the conditions in society which influence women's and men's health in order to be able to undertake preventive work as physicians." Some universities have included gender in their teaching goals, thus emphasising the need for integrating gender in all curricula at the university. There are examples of introducing gender sensitive practices within clinical medicine, for example, via teaching strategies for pelvic examination (Wijma & Dahlgren 1990). By using "professional" patients as teachers (as discussed by Robertson et al., this volume), medical students learn palpation techniques better than those who learn on actual patients.

Lessons Learnt

Below, I will summarise my lessons learned from ten years of teaching gender in the School of Medicine. First of all, it is important to be aware of the gender order in the classroom, that is, the gendered distribution of influence, power and space. Because of the gender order and the reactions that gender teaching provokes, it has proved useful to teach gender-related issues alone as a female teacher, but with a male colleague. Otherwise, there is a risk that male students will dominate the lessons by interruption, making irrelevant comments, questioning what is being said, and judging the woman instructor as a "biased feminist."

Second, it has proven valuable to relate gender teaching to the overall goals regarding gender in the curriculum, university regulations, and the regulation of higher education. Anchoring the subject within the university structures is one way of encouraging student engagement with the subject material.

Third, it is useful to identify the preconceived notions that students have in relation to the semantics of gender and feminism. A Swedish feminist researcher in organisational theory, Anna Wahl, has developed what she calls "the cloud," in order to catch these notions in gender education (1996). She starts her lessons with a simple question: "What do you think about when you hear the word feminism?" and then writes on the blackboard the associations from the students. From this free list, she identifies three main structures: words related to feminist politics, to feminist ideology and to feminist research. Above these main areas, a cloud floats filled with the preconceived notions of the students. The cloud can be identified and dismissed as irrelevant to the academic subject. Thereafter, the aim of the lecture should be identified: to deal with feminist research, not to take up feminist politics or ideologies. Feminist research needs to be emphasised as an academic field of knowledge, where popular conceptions and individual experiences have no place. This method is a tool that can help the students to articulate common beliefs around feminism and thus contribute to a teaching environment where knowledge-based research can be taught.

Fourth, teaching needs to be anchored in the students' reality. Rather than starting from the theoretical level, it has been useful to begin with clinically relevant examples, and then to introduce gendered interpretations and theoretical frameworks. Two useful clinical cases are violence against women and women with misunderstood symptoms. Violence against women constitutes a huge but neglected public health issue (Rönnberg & Hammarström 2000), and women with so-called diffuse symptoms constitute a large part of general practitioners' practices. Both subjects are often neglected in traditional medical education.

Fifth, make sure you use the best pedagogic measures so that the students do not have anything "technical" to complain about. This is of course difficult for teachers who are questioned and interrupted all the time.

Sixth, gender should not be taught only as a separate subject on the curriculum. Instead, gender research needs to be skillfully integrated into the whole curriculum, through various teaching opportunities throughout the course. Increased awareness of sex-related health, as well as biological differences between men and women, needs to be integrated in the whole curriculum.

Seventh and perhaps most important, there are risks in teaching gender. One risk is that the resistance among students towards gender teaching is so large, that students may only get negative experiences from your teaching. Another risk is that the teaching will only confirm students' stereotyped expectations regarding what they consider to be typically male or female behaviour or character. If the teaching only focuses on either descriptions of gender differences or on students' attitudes, without any gendered theoretical interpretation of findings or discussion of attitude, there is a risk that the students will increase their essentialist values. The risk of increased essentialism as a consequence of the teaching is of course greatest when teachers, without training in the gender theoretical field of knowledge, teach the subject. It is necessary therefore to integrate gender into the whole curriculum with care.

What could be done? Integrating gender throughout the curriculum, by teachers with good competence in gender issues, appears especially valuable. In order to broaden knowledge of gender issues, interested teachers could be offered special training courses within the subject, as well as continuous support from gender researchers to develop their teaching. The risks of gender teaching need to be discussed among all teachers in the subject. On the other hand, teaching about biological, differences between men and women (e.g., pharmacological or biochemical differences) can be taught without any knowledge in gender issues.

CONCLUSION

In this paper, I have analysed the experiences from the Nordic countries, especially Sweden, in relation to the integration of gender into research and teaching within the positivistic-dominated academic medicine. The prerequisite for developing gender research in medicine has been a grassroots movement of gender researchers with political support. Despite political support, the integration has not been easy. Academic medicine has responded to this development with different strategies such as resistance and redefining concepts.

Through example, I have argued that while academic medicine has willingly accepted state funding of women's studies/gender research, it has tried to transform the resources into something else, while combating gender issues related to power analysis and theoretical development.

Medical students' reactions to gender education can be compared with academic medicine's reactions towards gender research. Obstacles and possibilities (summarised as seven lessons learnt) are described in relation to teaching gender in schools of medicine. Most important is to recognise the risks for increased gender stereotypes and increased essentialism among the students, unless gender is taught from a theoretical perspective.

Gender research has been integrated slowly into both research and teaching within Nordic academic medicine, although the pathway has not been easy. So far, gender research has had strong political support, but while most political parties declare feminist sympathy, we can expect a backlash in relation to investments in gender research and teaching. But the more we manage to build before the political wind changes, the stronger our power of resistance.

REFERENCES

Ahlgren, C. and Hammarström, A. (1999). *Has the increased focus on vocational rehabilitation led to an increase in young employee's return to work after work-related disorders?* Scandinavian Journal of Public Health, 27, 220-227.

Alexanderson, K., Wingren, G. and Rosdahl, I. (1998). *Gender analyses of medical textbooks on dermatology, epidemiology, occupational medicine and public health.* Education for Health, 2, 151-163.

Alexandersson, K. (1999). *An assessment protocol for gender analysis of medical literature.* Women and Health, 29(2), 81-98.

Berliner, H. S. (1975). *A larger perspective on the Flexner report.* International Journal of Health Service, 4, 573-592.

Burger, W. (2001). *The relation between medical education and the medical profession's world view.* Medicine, Health Care and Philosophy, 4, 79-84.

Connell, R. W. (1987). *Gender and Power: Society, the Person and Sexual Politics.* Allen & Unwin, Sydney.

Connell, R. W. (2000). *The Men and the Boys.* Berkeley and Los Angeles Press: University of California Press.

Courtney, W. H. (2000). *Constructions of masculinity and their influence on men's well being: a theory of gender and health.* Social Science & Medicine, 50, 1385-1401.

Gustavsson, R. (1989). *Origins of authority: the organisation of medical care in Sweden.* International Journal of Health Service, 19(1), 121-133.

Hammarström, A. (1999). *Why feminism in public health? Editorial for a special issue on feminism in Public Health.* Scandinavian Journal of Public Health, 4, 241-244.

Hammarström, A. (2002). *The development of gender research within the medical academy.* Kvinnovetenskaplig tidskrift (in Swedish, English summary), 2-3, 93-113.

Hammarström, A., Härenstam, A. and Östlin, P. (2001). Gender and health: concepts and explanatory models. In P. Östlin et al. (eds): *Gender Inequalities in Health–an edited volume designed to explain the considerable differences in morbidity and mortality that can be observed between men and woman.* Harvard University Press, Harvard (pp. 1-22).

Lundgren, E. (1995). Feminist Theory and Violent Empiricism. In: *A Feminist Theory and Violent Empiricism.* Anonymous. Avebury: Aldershot.

Löfmark, U. and Hammarström, A. (2001). *How are sex differences discussed in research on revascularisation in coronary heart disease? A qualitative gender analysis.* Läkartidningen (in Swedish, English summary), 30, 3306-3312.

Macintyre, S., Hunt, K. and Sweeting, H. (1996). *Gender differences in health: are things really as simple as they seem?* Soc. Sci. Med, 42, 617-624.

Reviewers' opinion regarding the applicants to the professorship in general practice, with special focus on Women's Studies at Linköping University (1993). Official report 22 June.

Rubin, G. (1975). Traffic in women. In Reiter (ed): *Towards an Anthropology of Women.* London and New York: Monthly Review Press.

Rönnberg, A. K. and Hammarström, A. (2000). *Barriers encountered by women exposed to sexualised violence in their interactions with the health care system–a literature review.* Scand J Public Health, 28(3), 222-229.

Wahl, A. (1996). *The cloud–to teach about feminist research.* Kvinnovetenskaplig tidskrift (in Swedish, English summary), 3-4(17), 31-44.

Wennerås, C. and Wold, A. (1997). *Nepotism and sexism in peer-review.* Nature, 387, 341-343.

West, C. and Zimmerman, D. H. (1987). *Doing gender.* Gender & Society, 2, 125-151.

Wijma, B. and Dahlgren, L. O. (1990). *"Professional" patients teach students gynaecological palpation techniques.* Läkartidningen (in Swedish), 9, 645-647.

Index

Academic medicine, resistance and
    power to define in, 126-131
AMC. *See* Australian Medical Council
    (AMC)
*American Journal of Obstetrics &
    Gynecology*, 1
American Journal of Public Health,
    14,28,90
Anderson, D., 63
Anderson, M., 35
Anthropology, medical, clinical,
    teaching of, gendered
    perspective on, 23-34. *See
    also* Clinical medical
    anthropology, teaching of,
    gendered perspective on
Aspirin Study, 13
Attitude(s), lesbian-health,
    international education
    regarding, 95-96
Australia, medical schools in,
    recommendations for, 99-100
Australian College of Rural and
    Remote Medicine, 84
Australian Drug Foundation study,
    91-92
Australian Lesbian Medical
    Association, 93,95,98
Australian Medical Association, 91
Australian Medical Council (AMC), 97
Authority, of CTAs, 61

Bartoshuk, L.M., 12,14
Bauman, K.A., 95

Benoit, C., 30
Bickel, J., 2
Bishop, E., 24

Cartwright, E., 3,23
Cassell, J., 29
CDC. *See* Centers for Disease Control
    (CDC)
Centers for Disease Control (CDC), 13
Centers of Excellence in Women's
    Health, 13
Clinical medical anthropology,
    teaching of, gendered
    perspective on, 23-34
    conversation analysis in clinical
        setting, 26-27
    cultural construction of risk and
        stigmatized populations,
        27-29
    patients' stories, 25-26
Clinical teaching associates (CTAs),
    50
Clinical Teaching Associates (CTAs)
    in Gynaecology Program,
    53-60
    authority of, 61
    comfort of, 61
    cultural diversity among, 60-61
    establishment of, issues related to,
        60-62
    ethical considerations related to,
        61-62
    evaluation of, 57-60,59f,59t
    power of, 61
    recruitment of, 54-55

http://www.haworthpress.com/store/product.asp?sku=J013
© 2003 by The Haworth Press, Inc. All rights reserved.
10.1300/J013v37n04_10

relationships between, 60
self-esteem of, 61
training of, 55,56b-57b
in Victoria, 53-60,56b-57b,59f,59t
Clinician(s), genderizing
    understandings of, 29-31
Comfort, of CTAs, 61
Commonwealth Department of Health
    and Aged Care, General
    Practice Branch of, 70
Commonwealth Government, 84
Commonwealth Government of
    Australia, 68
Congressional Caucus for Women's
    Issues, 13
Connell, R.W., 123
Conversation analysis, in clinical
    setting, 26-27
Cosmopolitan, 16
Council of Scientific Affairs of the
    American Medical
    Association, 90
CTAs. *See also* Clinical teaching
    associates (CTAs)

Dessaix, R., 32
Diagnosis, foreknowledge and, 31-32

Education, medical. *See* Medical
    education
Eighth Annual Congress on Women's
    Health and Gender-Based
    Medicine, 19
Equal Rights Amendment (ERA), 13
ERA. *See* Equal Rights Amendment
    (ERA)
Ethical issues, in CTA Gynaecology
    program, 61-62

Faculty Curriculum Committee, 83
FDA. *See* Food and Drug
    Administration (FDA)
Flexner Report, 125

Flinders University, 98
Fonda, J., 19
Fonn, S., 105
Food and Drug Administration (FDA),
    13
Foreknowledge, diagnosis and, 31-32
Francois-Xavier Bagnoud Centre for
    Health and Human Rights, of
    Harvard School of Public
    Health, 108

Gay and Lesbian Association of
    Doctors and Dentists
    (GLADD) workshop, 94-95
Gay and Lesbian Medical Association,
    92-93
Gender
    defined, 123
    in medical curricula, 35-47. *See
        also* Gender-issues
        perspective in medicine, in
        Sweden, course organizer
        views of
    rural case study, 67-87
        evaluation of, 77-81,78t,
            80t-83t
        facilitative environment in,
            68-70
        framework of, 72-73
        students in, 71-72
        teaching curriculum in, 73-77
        workforce in, 69-70
    testing of, legitimacy of, 83-84
    in medical research and education,
        121-133
        development of, 122-126
        introduction to, 122
        from periphery to centre,
            125-126
        political investments in, 126
        from women's studies to,
            122-124
    in medicine, teaching of, 128-130

research on, *vs.* research on
women's health, 124-125
Gender and Society, 14
Gender equality, health care
practitioners in, 105-120. *See
also* Health care practitioners,
role in gender equality
Gender issues, learning about, 41,42t-43t
Gender Issues for Rural Doctors, 68
Gender Working Party, 83
Gender-issues perspective in medicine,
in Sweden, course organizer
views of, 35-47
study of
contribution to knowledge,
38-40,39t-40t
discussion, 44-46
follow-up seminar, 42,44
implementation in teaching,
40-41,42t
improving teaching, 42
introduction to, 36-37
method in, 37-38,38t
results of, 38-44,38t-40t,42t-44t
General Accounting Office, 13
General Medical Council (GMC), 95
General Practice Branch, of
Commonwealth Department
of Health and Aged Care, 70
GLADD workshop. *See* Gay and
Lesbian Association of
Doctors and Dentists
(GLADD) workshop
GMC. *See* General Medical Council
(GMC)
Goffman, E., 29
Goldstein, M.Z., 1
Goteborg University, 4
Government, priorities of, transformation
of, 126-127
GTA instructional method, 52-53
Gunn, J., 49
Gynaecology Teaching Associate
(GTA) instructional method,
52-53

Gynecology Teaching Associate
programs, 4,5

Hale, F.A., 95
Hammarstrom, A., 7,121
Harrison, J., 91
Harvard School of Public Health,
Francois-Xavier Bagnoud
Centre for Health and Human
Rights of, 108
Haseltine, F., 14
Health care, quality, for lesbians,
barriers to, 92-93
Health care practitioners, role in
gender equality, 105-120
courses related to, 108-112
dealing with relationship aspects
by, 112-117
impact of, 117-118
participants in, 108-112
Health Workers for Change, 116,118
Health Workers for Choice, 116
Healy, B., 13
Hegarty, K., 49
Henderson, P., 95
Henrich, J.B., 3,11,12,14

ICPD, 110
Idaho State University, 4
Institute of Medicine, 90
Intersex Society of North America
(ISNA), 18
IOM. *See* Institute of Medicine
ISNA. *See* Intersex Society of North
America (ISNA)

JAMA. *See Journal of the American
Medical Association (JAMA)*
Jefferson, G., 27
Johnson, M.H., 95
*Journal of the American Medical
Association (JAMA)*, 14

Journal of Women's Health, 14
Journal of Women's Health and
    Gender-Based Medicine, 14,19

Lee, J., 63
Lesbian, gay, bisexual and transgender
    (LGBT) perspectives, 28
Lesbian(s), quality health care for,
    barriers to, 92-93
Lesbian health
    attitudes toward, international
        education regarding, 95-96
    knowledge of, 91-92
    in medical education, in Australia,
        97-99
    outing of, in medical education,
        89-103
    introduction to, 90-91
Lesbian health issues, medical
        education regarding, 96-97
Lesbian medical students and doctors,
        marginalization of, medical
        attitudes leading to, 93-94
Levitt, L., 69
LGBT perspectives, 28
Linkoping University, 129
Lockhart, H., 63
Lorber, J., 18
Louisiana State University, 96

Manderson, L., 1
McEwin, K., 69
McNair, R., 6,89
Medical anthropology, clinical,
    teaching of, gendered
    perspective on, 23-34. *See*
    also Clinical medical
    anthropology, teaching of,
    gendered perspective on
Medical curriculum(a)
    gender and, rural case study, 67-87.
        See also Gender, and medical
        curriculum, rural case study

gender in, 35-47. *See also*
    Gender-issues perspective in
    medicine, in Sweden, course
    organizer views of
Medical education
    in Australia, lesbian health–related,
        97-99
    gender in, 121-133. *See also*
        Gender, in medical research
        and education
    lesbian health issues–related, 96-97
    outing lesbian health in, 89-103.
        See also Lesbian health,
        outing of, in medical
        education
    regarding lesbian health attitudes,
        95-96
Medical Faculty of Goteborg
    University, 36,37
Medical research, gender in, 121-133.
    See also Gender, in medical
    research and education
Medical Research Council (MRC),
    125,127-128
Medical schools, in Australia,
    recommendations for, 99-100
Medical Women's International
    Association, 84
Medicine, women and men in, 68-69
Mega-Dose, 16,19
Monash University, 53,68,71
    outcome at, 81,83
    Rural General Practice Education
        at, 73
    Rural Practice Association at, 72
Monash University School of Rural
    Health, 84
MRC. *See* Medical Research Council
    (MRC)
MTV, 16,19

Nagle, C., 63
National Institutes of Health (NIH), 6

Office of Research on Women's
  Health of, 16
National Organization for Women
  (NOW), 18
New England Journal of Medicine, 14
New York Times, 14
Night Letter, 32
NIH. *See* National Institutes of Health
  (NIH)
NIH's Office of Research on Women's
  Health, 16
Ninth Annual Congress on Women's
  Health and Gender-Based
  Medicine, 19
NOW. *See* National Organization for
  Women (NOW)

O'Connor, V., 49
Office of Research on Women's
  Health, 13
  of NIH, 16
Our Bodies, Our Selves, 3,16

Pap testing, sensitive
  characteristics of, 52
  teaching of, need for, 51-52
PapScreen Victoria, 53,62-63
Parliamentary Assembly of the
  Council of Europe, 90
Physician's Health Study, 13
Planned Parenthood, 17
Population(s), stigmatized, cultural
  construction of, 27-29
Power, of CTAs, 61
Professor of Rural Health, 72
Public Health Service, 13

Quality health care, for lesbians,
  barriers to, 92-93
Queensland Cancer Fund, 53
Queensland University, 51

Ragone, H., 31
Rice, K., 63
Risk, cultural construction of, 27-29
Robb, N., 97
Robertson, K., 5,49
Rogers, N., 3,11,14,18
Rourke, J., 70
Royal Women's Hospital, 98
Rural General Practice Education, at
  Monash University, 73
Rural Practice Association, at Monash
  University, 72
Rural Undergraduate Support and
  Coordination (RUSC)
  program, 70,71

Sacks, H., 27
Sandall, J., 30
Schegeloff, E., 27
School of Public Health, at University
  of the Witwatersrand,
  Johannesburg, 106
Scientific Council of Medicine (SCM),
  128
SCM. *See* Scientific Council of
  Medicine (SCM)
Seaman, B., 17-18
Searle, J., 45
Self-esteem, of CTAs, 61
"Sex," defined, 123
Sexuality minorities, within medicine,
  well-being of, methods for
  improving, 94-95
Shelley, D., 7
Society for the Advancement of
  Women's Health Research,
  14
Soderstrom, M., 35
South Australian Department of
  Human Services, 91
Stevens, P.E., 93
Strasser, R., 70
Swedish Freedom of the Press Act,
  127

Swedish Government, 128
Swedish Regulation of Higher
	Education, 129

Teaching Gendered Medicine, 84
The Royal Women's Hospital,
	Melbourne, 93
Tolhurst, H., 70
Twine, F., 31

Undergraduate Rural Curriculum
	Conference, 70,71
University of Adelaide, 99
University of Cambridge, 96
University of Florida, Women's
	Studies Center at, 14
University of Illinois, at Chicago, 14
University of Maryland, 14
University of Melbourne,
	5,51,53,57-58,63,71,98
University of Melbourne Rural
	General Practitioner Teacher
	Training, 73
University of Newcastle, 98
University of Queensland,
	5,53,54,57-58,98
University of Witwatersrand, South
	Africa, Women's Health
	Project of, 6

VA. *See* Veterans Administration (VA)
Veterans Administration (VA), 13
Victorian Ministerial Advisory
	Committee on Gay and
	Lesbian Health, 91

Wahl, A., 130
Wainer, J., 5-6,67
Well Woman Check, clinical teaching
	associate program for,
	establishment of, 49-65

study of, 50-51
	background of, 51-53
Well-being, of sexuality minorities
	within medicine, methods for
	improving, 94-95
Wenneras, C., 127,128
Westerstahl, A., 4,35
WHO. *See* World Health Organization
	(WHO)
WHP. *See* Women's Health Project
	(WHP)
Wold, A., 127,128
Women and Health, 14
Women in Medicine, 84
Women in Rural Practice, 84
Women's and Gender Studies
	Program, 3,15
Women's Feelings and Issues, 17
Women's health
	research on, *vs.* research on gender,
		124-125
	teaching of, into 21st century, 11-21
	women teaching, issues in
		establishment of clinical
		teaching associate program
		for Well Woman Check,
		49-65. *See also* Well Woman
		Check, clinical teaching
		associate program for
Women's Health and Wellbeing
	consultation paper, 91
Women's Health and Wellbeing
	policy, 90-91
Women's Health Initiative, 13,18
Women's Health Issues, 14,19
Women's Health Project (WHP), 106
	of University of Witwatersrand,
		South Africa, 6
Women's Health Project, School of
	Public Health, Johannesburg,
	South Africa, 105,106
Women's Studies Center, at University
	of Florida, 14
WONCA. *See* World Organisation of
	Family Doctors (WONCA)

World Health Organization (WHO), 108

World Organisation of Family Doctors (WONCA), 84

Wrede, S., 30

Yale Medical School, 12

Yale University, 11,12

Yale University School of Medicine, 3

Yale Women's Health course, 11,12

You Don't Know Dick, 29

Zelek, B., 44-45